Man, Cancer and Immunity

Man, Cancer and Immunity

ALISTAIR J. COCHRAN, M.D.

Reader in Pathology
University Department of Pathology
Western Infirmary, Glasgow

1978

ACADEMIC PRESS

London   New York   San Francisco

A Subsidiary of Harcourt Brace Jovanovich, Publishers

ACADEMIC PRESS INC. (LONDON) LTD.
24/28 Oval Road
London NW1

United States Edition published by
ACADEMIC PRESS INC.
111 Fifth Avenue
New York, New York 10003

Copyright © 1978 by
ACADEMIC PRESS (INC.) LONDON LTD.

Library of Congress Catalog Card Number: 78-52087
ISBN: 0-12-177550-X

PRINTED IN GREAT BRITAIN BY THE LAVENHAM PRESS LIMITED
LAVENHAM SUFFOLK

Foreword

by Georg Klein

This book is a balanced report of the widely different views of tumour immunology which while not partisan is nevertheless committed. It does not cover everything published in the field of human tumour immunology in recent years, although it covers most of the relevant studies. It emphasizes that while a variety of host responses have been shown to act against human tumours not all of them are necessarily immunological. The author gives a good appraisal of experimental tumour immunology, yet stresses the impossibility of directly translating animal studies to man. Since the book is primarily written for clinicians, it rightly emphasizes that the lack of a total understanding of the mechanisms of biological phenomena does not exclude the possibility that some of the phenomena may find applications in the diagnosis and/or the follow up of cancer patients prior to the development of an appreciation of their biological significance.

Appropriately, the book starts from the clinical observations which have shown sporadically, anecdotally, but imperiously and persistently that host responses exist against human tumours. It is made clear that modern developments in this area started by the unequivocal demonstration that some animal tumours are immunogenic in the hosts in which they arise. This is particularly true for chemically and virally induced tumours, and much less so, or not so for spontaneous tumours. The increasing complexity of the "immunological orchestra" is emphasized and it is made clear that results obtained in a given system cannot be translated to any other. By implication, *human tumour immunology must be based on direct enquiries into the human system itself.*

The history of tumour immunology is characterized by many ups and downs. Early enthusiasm about the possibility of protection by immunization, based on results obtained in studies of long transplanted tumours was replaced by complete pessimism when it became clear that the reactions detected were directed against transplantation antigens rather than antigens unique to the tumours. In the early 1960s tumour associated or tumour specific transplantation antigens were discovered on chemically and virally induced tumours. Since these antigens were capable of inducing rejection reactions in critically syngeneic or even in autologous hosts, a second wave of enthusiasm was generated for studies of immunology. The concept that some tumours contained unique antigenic molecules gained surprisingly rapid acceptance in view of the considerable volume of earlier negative studies. It is even more surprising that there followed sweeping generalizations postulating that *all* animal and human tumours were probably antigenic. Although voices of warning against the uncritical acceptance of such generalization have not been lacking, they have been largely ignored sometimes even by those who did the relevant experiments but who have been subsequently carried away by the optimistic spirit of the times. Yet, there is increasing evidence that not all tumours are necessarily recognized by the immune responses of the host. And why should they be? Virus-induced tumours bear the same surface-associated antigen, as long as they are produced by the same virus. In this special situation surveillance has a clear target to focus on and, in the cases where the species had previous extensive contact with the virus, is aided by an immense prehistory of natural selection.

Spontaneous tumours seem likely to represent a very different situation. These are tumours which arise without experimental interference and emerge at the end of a prolonged progression which is now understood to be the gradual evolution of cellular independence from a variety of local and general restrictive influences including hormonal and, no doubt, immunological factors. If tumour associated antigens do arise in slow-developing spontaneous tumours it would be expected that they would meet a strong selective pressure resulting in low immunogenic or non-immunogenic tumours, in contrast to the rapidly developing tumours induced by strong chemical carcinogens or powerful oncogenic viruses.

The question whether all potential tumour cells are recognized by the immune response and tumour outgrowth is a matter of subsequent breakdown of such responses or, alternatively, whether there has been an absence of recognition *ab initio*, not because tumour cells do not differ in membrane and other properties, but because their own micro-evolution (progression) has moulded them into a chameleon-like non-recognisability by the Ir (immune responsiveness) gene equipment of the host, is not merely of academic interest. Obviously, both experimental and practical measures will have to be quite different in the two situations outlined. In the former case, the problem is how to correct a malfunctioning response, in the latter, how to induce the host to recognize neoplasia associated membrane changes which are not spontaneously antigenic.

It is easy to be disappointed by the lack of progress in tumour immunology and the lack of major technological advances applicable in the clinic. This reaction, however, is in large measure a result of the quite unreasonable levels of expectation engendered by the intense pressures developed by the anxiety of clinicians, laymen, research administrators and politicians to apply laboratory results to patient management with minimal delay. These pressures, in addition to overheating our levels of expectation are counter productive by endangering the traditional and well founded "gradualism" by which the advance of scientific knowledge occurs. Specifically accelerated speculation leads to erroneous concepts and the uncritical and unnecessarily prolonged investigation of such concepts, which in turn perpetuates central fallacies and myths.

Tumour immunology certainly has its share of middle-aged and elderly myths but there are some indications that these are now being recognised for what they are and that the subject is presently proceeding on a more strengthened scientific basis. The main priority remains the generation in a variety of laboratories of that scientific atmosphere without which progress is impossible and which permits the generation and *recognition* of the significant unexpected spin off result. Obviously we are at the *very beginning* of this whole game and have *barely scratched its surface.* I would compare the present situation in tumour immunology to the first developments of the H-2 field or the earliest recognition of transplantation antigens by the use of inbred strains. Manipulating the immune response in favour of the cancer patient may or may not be feasible, but we are unlikely to know this answer in the short term.

This book is a timely review of the many strands of evidence which point to a host-response to cancer, and of the initial experimental attempts to investigate this interesting phenomenon. It provides a readable account of the somewhat shaky foundations on which a more rigidly scientific discipline of tumour immunology could be erected.

Stockholm
April 1978

For Janie, Angus and Sara

Preface

My early research activities, begun at the suggestion of the late Professor D. F. Cappell, were concerned with clinicopathological factors which related to the death or survival of patients with malignant melanoma. The results of these studies made it clear that the outcome in this situation depended on numerous characteristics of the tumour cells and the patient and the manner in which patient and tumour interacted. The realisation that there were host reactions to tumour cells came at a time of expanding interest in the role of immunity in many different diseases including cancer. I have therefore spent much of the last ten years thinking about and investigating immunity and tumours in animals and man and remain convinced that host responses, including immune reactions, play an important part in the control of tumour development and spread. This notion is widely shared although, with the passage of time, it has become increasingly clear that the involvement of immune factors in malignant disease is complex and subtle.

Discussion with colleagues who are not immediately involved in research into tumour immunology has made it clear that the subject is one about which many would wish to be better informed. However, the voluminous literature on tumour-related immunology and relatively complex technical jargon of the immunologist make it difficult for the general reader to obtain a balanced viewpoint. This seems especially a problem for individuals who graduated before the new wave of immunology had broken on medical and general science courses. This monograph attempts to provide a general account of the major principles of tumour immunity and an attempt has been made to limit the content of jargon and where this has proved impossible to explain in a relatively simple manner the terms used. This was the initial intention and if I have failed in this aim I must ask my readers to, as far as possible, take the thought for the deed. I have concentrated on the situation in man and discuss animal findings only when this is necessary to support a concept, or where human studies are lacking. The subject and its literature proliferate at a frightening pace and the subject matter, while as up to date as I could make it in the Autumn of 1977, will certainly be out of date in parts by the time of publication. It should, however, provide a relatively stable platform from which the reader may venture into specific areas of the subsequent literature.

My views have been very much influenced by contact and discussion with many physicians and scientists in the United Kingdom and many other parts of the world. These contacts have been invaluable and it is my sincere hope that this source of intellectual stimulation will continue to remain available to me. I have received immense support and stimulus from Professor J. R. Anderson of this Department and Professors Eva and Georg Klein of the Department of Tumor Biology, Karolinska Institute, Stockholm. I have had the good fortune to collaborate with and receive the friendship of many stimulating colleagues including Drs. Peter Gunvén, Jan Stjernswärd, Francis Wiener, Rolf Kiessling, Bal Gothoskar and Ulrich Jehn in Sweden and Professors Donald Morton, Wallace Clark, Sidney Golub, Leon Rosenberg, Herbert Wohl and Max Essex in the United States. My work in Glasgow has been made possible by invaluable associations with Professor Rona Mackie, Drs. Walter Spilg, Catherine Ross, Robert Grant and Alan Jackson, Ms. Deirdre Hoyle, Lindsay Morrison and Gaye Todd. As most of the original studies described have involved patients these would have been impossible without the kindness of many clinical colleagues who permitted me to study their patients in the Karolinska Sjukhuset, Stockholm, The Western Infirmary, Gartnavel General Hospital, The Royal Infirmary, The West of Scotland Regional Plastic Surgery Centre at Canniesburn Hospital, The West of Scotland Regional Radiotherapy and Oncology Service, Stobhill General Hospital, The Victoria Infirmary, The Royal Hospital for Sick Children, The Southern General Hospital and Hairmyres Hospital.

The production of the book has involved many people and it is a pleasure to be able to thank them publicly. Mrs. Maureen Ralston skilfully and patiently typed the book in draft and final form. Photographs were kindly provided by Professor Tom Gibson (Fig. 2.2), Professor Rona Mackie (Fig. 2.3), Dr. Gavin Sandilands (Fig. 6.1), and Dr. Robert Grant (Fig. 8.6). Mr. Peter Kerrigan advised on photography and helped in many practical ways. Mr. Robin Callender arranged for the production of the line drawings. The book was read at various stages by Professor J. R. Anderson, Dr. Andrew Sandison, Dr. Geoffrey Clements, Dr. Alan Jackson and Professor Rona Mackie from all of whom much sage counsel was received. I am indebted to Professor Georg Klein for his foreword which provides such an excellent beginning to the book.

My wife and children patiently supported me during the gestation period of the book and valiantly bore with any slight increment in my grumpiness and my greater than usual obsession with the laboratory.

Glasgow   *July 1978*

Contents

1

Introduction

Cancer commands more interest than ever before in virtually all sections of the community. This disease, which is a major cause of death in adults in the developed countries, has generated interest, emotion and fear which used to be the province of infectious disease in general and tuberculosis in particular. Interest is not confined solely to the medical and allied professions, but is high in governmental and international agencies concerned with health care. The public at large is increasingly aware of and informed about the nature and problems of malignant disease. This increasing general awareness of cancer is partly the result and partly the cause of the increased coverage of malignant disease in publications available to the general public. The upsurge in interest has brought benefits in the form of increased governmental support of cancer research, the emergence of oncology as a new clinical speciality and the development of multi-disciplinary centres of excellence where accumulated experience from referred patients permits optimum treatment of relatively rare cancers. Not least among these benefits is the gradual acceptance by the public that cancer is, like other human ailments, to some degree explicable on the basis of orthodox theories of pathology and clinical medicine and is, in its early stages, at least relatively responsive to well-established forms of therapy.

The translation of cancer from an abstruse medical concept to a subject widely discussed and well understood by a proportion of the lay public presents new problems to physicians dealing with the informed cancer patient or the relatives of such patients. Sources of cancer information are now very different from the blandly non-committal entries of "Home Doctor" books and "Domestic Medical Encyclopaedias" and range from the deliberately diffuse replies of correspondents who answer medical questions in local and national newspapers to the very precisely detailed and generally accurate accounts of specific cancers and of aspects of cancer treatment and research which appear from time to time in high circulation periodicals, on radio and in television documentaries.

The practitioner may expect to encounter patients who are informed, not only about the nature, significance and prognosis of a particular cancer, but also about growth areas in developmental cancer therapy and experimental cancer research. Regardless of the extent of their own expertise patients reasonably expect that their physicians will be able to give a valid opinion on the many facets of their disease and its treatment. This can present real problems, especially in areas such as radiation biology, the pharmacology of chemotherapy, multiple agent chemotherapy, the relationship of viruses to cancer, the molecular biology of cancer and immunological aspects of cancer where there have been recent and rapid developments. This book is intended to give a general account of the last topic and it is hoped that it will help the reader to appreciate the extent, nature and significance of immune reactions which develop in response to cancer cells. I have also attempted to indicate those areas where immunology may be exploited to assist in cancer diagnosis and in the management of patients with malignant disease.

That cancers which appear identical on cytological, histological, histochemical and functional grounds behave quite differently in terms of local growth and speed and extent of distant spread in different patients is the everyday experience of those involved in the clinical care of cancer patients. This is really not a surprising observation and depends upon variables relating to the patient, characteristics of the tumour cells and on an equally wide range of variation in the reaction of the tumour bearing host to the tumour. The nature, extent and biological significance of this reaction not only differs from patient to patient, but also changes within the same patient as the tumour progresses or regresses. The reaction may also alter as a result of anti-tumour therapy, intercurrent disease and treatment directed to coexisting conditions unrelated to the cancer.

Many different characteristics of a cell dictate whether it will survive or not within the relatively demanding environment of the human body. It is likely that all cells are subjected to a detailed and continuing scrutiny and that only cells possessed of certain clearly defined and quite remarkable characteristics survive. The mechanisms involved in this scrutiny are certainly complex and involve many known body systems such as the macrophages, cells of the lymphocyte series, mast cells, neutrophils, basophils, eosinophils and the complex humoral molecules of the inflammatory mechanisms. These are known factors but it is equally possible that other as yet unidentified types of cell-cell interaction and mutual identification are involved and it is possible that the systems so far identified are relatively unimportant in the identification and control of deleterious mutants, including potential and actual cancer cells. Be this as it may, much interest has focused on the role of immunology in cancer. This is partly because this system is slightly better understood than most others and the classical and fruitful studies of the immunology of infectious disease, blood transfusion, auto-immune disease and organ transplantation have made available a multiplicity of techniques for immunological studies, *in vitro* and *in vivo*. The very multiplicity of techniques which has been developed reflects the lack of simply executed, reliable immunological assays of cell-mediated and humoral immunity which can readily be correlated with significant clinical events. It is salutary that immunological tests do not always distinguish sharply between patients with limited primary cancer and those with more advanced disease; a distinction which is all too readily made in the majority of cancer patients by the simplest clinical investigations.

Immunological study of cancer patients nonetheless offers a variety of highly desirable prospects. At a clinical level the identification of tumour products, including tumour associated antigens, offers the prospect of relatively simple screening tests for the identification of early cancers. A simple and reliable approach of this kind which does not involve expensive equipment or surgical intervention would permit the repeated examination of high risk groups, with the prospect of early diagnosis. Serial monitoring of patients after excision of a primary tumour is already practicable, employing the repeated assessment of blood levels of tumour markers and products such as human chorionic gonadotrophins, carcino-embryonic antigen and alpha-fetoprotein. Increasing levels of these materials predict the development of recurrences and metastases before they become clinically detectable, which permits the early introduction of aggressive adjuvant therapy. Such products are available for only a limited number of tumours and may never become available for all tumours. Where tumour markers are not available a possible alternative approach is the detection and serial quantification of the strength of tumour-directed immune responses, as manifested by anti-tumour antibodies and lymphocytes sensitised to tumour associated antigens.

Immunologically based tumour diagnosis and patient monitoring seem real and reasonably immediate prospects. The "holy grail" of the cancer immunologist, however, is the development of immunological techniques for the prevention or treatment of cancer. Such techniques would ideally develop from a deeper understanding of the biology and immunology of cancer. Regrettably, this desirable level of understanding seems distinctly remote and this associated with the massive scale of the social, economic and clinical problems which result from the high incidence of cancer has prompted many pragmatic and possibly premature attempts at immunotherapy of cancer in man. In defence of this pragmatism it should, however, be realised that medicine abounds in examples of highly successful therapeutic approaches which preceded an understanding of their biological basis by many years.

It is of course possible that the high hopes for cancer diagnosis, patient monitoring and cancer treatment by immunological means may come to naught. Alternative and more efficient techniques employing quite separate approaches may be developed contemporaneously with or in succession to the immunological approaches. Whether this occurs or not it seems very probable that the present extensive efforts to study immunological aspects of cancer will achieve some advance in our basic understanding of cancer. And this, of itself, will be a worthwhile result and may provide a more advanced platform from which future and perhaps definitive studies may be mounted.

2

Clinical Observations Suggestive of a Host Response

The active investigation of tumour immunity employing immunisation and subsequent challenge by transplantation of tumour cells, a basic and highly productive approach used extensively in animal studies, has been severely limited in man by ethical considerations. As a result of this there has developed a very extensive literature on the application of *in vitro* tests to the study of tumour related and general immune reactions in cancer patients. This records numerous interesting phenomena, some of which mirror the results obtained in animals, but all presenting the major problem, that their relevance to events *in vivo* is difficult to assess. Such an assessment usually necessitates complex and time-consuming serial studies of moderately large numbers of patients to permit analysis of the role of factors such as advancing or regressing tumour, the various forms of treatment employed and intercurrent non-malignant disease. A substantial part of this book is concerned with an account of such *in vitro* phenomena. However, before undertaking an analysis of the clinical relevance of such contrived observations, it seems appropriate to search for clinical evidence of host defensive factors active against malignant disease. Nature's experiments have yielded much interesting information to the discerning eye in other clinical situations and have often indicated those areas in which laboratory investigations are most likely to be productive.

Immunological Surveillance

The most obvious function of the immunological system is to recognise and respond to foreign materials introduced into the body and to contain them by the production of specifically reactive antibody molecules and specifically sensitised lymphocytes, or to accept them by specific tolerance. The most obvious sources of such foreign antigens are micro-organisms and ingested or inhaled materials. It has however been argued that in addition to these gross responses there is a more subtle continuous "policing" of the body by roving macrophages and lymphocytes (immunological surveillance) which identify and react with any foreign "non-self" antigens encountered (Thomas, 1959; Burnet, 1967, 1970). In this way, in addition to microbial antigens and antigens on inanimate materials introduced by nose or mouth, endogenous host cells which develop an altered antigenic profile, either "spontaneously" or as a result of the action of micro-organisms or chemicals after the period of self-recognition and its associated tolerance (which ends at or around birth) will be identified as foreign and evoke an immune response. Burnet's suggestion is that cells recognisable as immunologically foreign, are identified and destroyed by the immune system. On the basis of what is known about the antigenicity of tumour cells (Chapter 4) it seems likely that mutant clones, including those with actual or potential malignant characteristics, would be susceptible to this type of immunological control. This concept has been a tremendous stimulus to thought and experiment in tumour immunology, but in the light of accumulating experimental and clinical observation certainly requires some modification (Prehn and Lappé, 1971).

If the immune surveillance theory, as originally conceived, is correct, it is predictable that individuals who have an inherited or acquired deficiency of their immunological apparatus will be more likely to develop cancer than are immunologically intact individuals. This is, to a limited extent, true. However, the increased frequency of tumours in the immunologically abnormal does not reflect the incidence of tumour types seen in the general population, there being a preponderance of tumours of the lymphoid system. This single observation makes it difficult to accept the original concept of general immunological surveillance as a means of controlling the development of tumours of all the various organ-systems. There are certainly dissatisfied critics of the unqualified acceptance of immune surveillance as a major or universally active process limiting tumour development. These critics base their concern on the low immunogenicity of most spontaneous tumours in animals and of tumours induced *in vitro* (Prehn, 1970), the fact that small numbers of highly antigenic tumour cells can thrive *in vivo* ("sneaking through") (Humphreys *et al.*, 1962; Potter *et al.*, 1969) where larger numbers are eliminated and the relatively small and generally unrepresentative increase in tumours in immunologically crippled animals and immunologically abnormal humans. The proponents of immune surveillance, however, claim that the clinically detectable tumour is the exception which proves the rule, that strongly antigenic tumours are destroyed when at a single cell stage or of very small size. This is a difficult argument to counter, although the capacity of small numbers of some strongly antigenic tumours to avoid immunological attack by sneaking through is worrying in this context. Prehn (1971, 1972) has gone further and by drawing an analogy between the behaviour of foetuses and tumours, both in a sense allografts, and by his own animal studies and interpreting those of others, makes a considerable case for the possibility that a weak immune response, or one which is impeded by, for instance, blocking "antibody" may actually increase tumour growth where a basically strong or unimpeded response will inhibit such growth. The latter situation, which would represent immune surveillance in its original sense, is in Prehn's view a much less frequent occurrence than the former.

Schwartz (1972) proposed an interesting hypothesis in which he attempted to link the classical immune surveillance ideas and a new immunoregulatory concept. From a basic observation that latent viruses in mouse lymphocytes could be activated by the graft-versus-host reaction *in vivo* and by a mixed lymphocyte culture reaction *in vitro* he hypothesised that immune reactions in man, be they to microorganisms, autoantigens, tumour associated antigens or the transplantation antigens of allografts might induce a similar viral activation. This was considered especially possible where the immune reaction was abnormal as a result of partial or total failure of the normal humoral or lymphocytic immunoregulatory mechanism, as might occur in an inherently abnormal immunological system, or one which had been rendered abnormal by, for instance, chemotherapy. He ingeniously linked this concept of aberrant immunoregulation with the classical theory by suggesting that virus transformed clones induced by the abnormally regulated immune response might have a selective survival advantage in the face of concurrently depressed surveillance. Laroye (1973) suggests that each individual is able to respond to a finite number of antigenic determinants and has thus a specific genetically programmed unresponsiveness to a (probably large) number of antigens. If the individual encounters such an antigen, no immune response would result, and if the antigen were a tumour-associated antigen tumour growth would result. This would then be seen as a failure of immune surveillance, which it is, although of an inherited rather than an acquired type.

The role and significance of immune surveillance thus remains unsettled. Animal experimentation and circumstantial evidence from appropriate human situations of inherited and acquired immune deficiency appear to support the prediction that the immunologically subnormal will have an increased incidence of tumours, although the situation is clearly more complex than would be the case if "immunological surveillance" and the development of malignancy interacted in the manner initially conceived.

Inherited Immunological Deficiency Conditions

Most severe immunological deficiency syndromes are incompatible with pro-longed survival, and in the absence of any means of prolonging life in those affected, it cannot be known whether such individuals are at greater than average risk of developing malignant disease. There are, however, a few such conditions such as infantile sex-linked agammaglobulinaemia (Bruton-type B cell deficiency), thymic hypoplasia (Di-George Syndrome of T cell deficiency) and severe combined deficiency (Swiss-type stem cell deficiency) which are compatible with survival for some years, survival which has been extended in recent years by attempts at immunological replacement therapy. These individuals have indeed been found to have an above average risk of developing malignant disease, although the risk appears to be essentially confined to the development of lymphomas and leukaemias rather than the cancers which affect immunologically normal individuals (Epstein *et al.*, 1966; Huber, 1968; Gatti and Good, 1971). The selective involvement of lymphoid tissues suggests that the disordered lymphoid system is more susceptible to carcinogenesis or permits the development of carcinogens which selectively act against it. The findings are clearly not those which would be expected if a surveillance apparatus covering a multiplicity of carcinogen exposed tissues was in abeyance.

Cancer Incidence and Age

If one excludes the small peak of malignant disease in the very young, due perhaps to anomalies of development or excessive carcinogen sensitivity of immature tissues and possibly viral factors in the acute leukaemias, the great majority of cancers develop in the older members of the population. The most common explanation of this observation is that carcinogen exposure, in terms of the amount of exposure to each individual carcinogen and the variety of carcinogens encountered, is cumulative and that time is necessary for this cumulated effect to induce malignancy in target tissues. This is certainly in line with what is known, from animal experiments, of threshold doses, single agent carcinogenesis, syncarcinogenesis and cocarcinogenesis. It is also accepted that after tissues have been exposed to a threshold dose of a carcinogen, a fixed time, the *latent period of carcinogenesis*, is necessary for the development of a detectable tumour. This is relatively fixed for each combination of carcinogen and species and reflects the time needed for the various steps which convert a normal cell to a malignant one and the time involved in amplification of the malignant clone to a clinically detectable mass. Even in experimental systems this process may occupy a considerable part of the animal's natural lifespan and may dictate the development of most human cancers later in life.

Important as the factors discussed above undoubtedly are, it has to be considered whether other changes associated with advancing age may increase susceptibility to carcinogenesis, or permit the escape from control and relatively unimpeded growth of mutant malignant clones. Many different factors such as hormonal alterations, nutritional deficiency and reduced rates of cell turnover may be involved, but it seems appropriate to confine the current consideration of this situation to the possibility that a decline of immune reactivity in the elderly may be significant. There is evidence that both humoral immunity (Wigzell and Stjernswärd, 1966; Kishimoto et al., 1969) and cell mediated immunity (Stjernswärd, 1966; Kishimoto et al., 1974) decline in mice with advancing age and that this decline is more frequent and earlier in mice prone to auto-immune disease (Stutman et al., 1968; Cantor et al., 1970; Rodey et al., 1971). Available data in man are very limited. A reduction in skin delayed hypersensitivity to recall antigens has been reported as occurring with ageing (Weber and Schlaeger, 1969; Serrou et al., 1974) and diminished in vitro lymphocyte blastogenesis on exposure to PHA is also on record (Hallgren and Wood, 1972). Chan, working in this Department, has found an age-related decline in BCG-induced leucocyte migration inhibition in tuberculin sensitive individuals (to be published). By contrast Rowley and McKay (1969) found no decline in responsiveness to salmonella flagellin, but it is possible that they were detecting a secondary response, and in animals such responses are less age dependent than the primary response (Morton and Siegel, 1968). Less direct evidence, if not of a decline in immune reactivity at least of a loss of fine control of immunological homeostasis by virtue of loss of self tolerance or aberration of specific suppressor activity, comes from the increasing incidence of autoantibodies with age (Walford, 1969; Whittingham et al., 1969; McKay, 1972) and the increase of amyloidosis in the elderly (Walford, 1974). It has even been reported that during a limited duration study of a single community a majority of those who died had autoantibodies, and that, after vascular disease, cancer was the commonest cause of death in the autoantibody positive group (McKay, 1972).

The evidence of the coexistence of declining immunological activity, and increasing cancer incidence with ageing is reasonably acceptable, however there is little or no evidence that the relationship is one of cause and effect. In view of the importance of this point further studies are urgently required.

An interesting philosophical point has been raised concerning the apparently poor capacity of the elderly to eradicate cancer. It has been suggested that, as those beyond the reproductive phase of life no longer serve a clear biological function in relation to species survival there has been no evolutionary development of an efficient mechanism for the control of spontaneous malignancy. This may be true, but even in the face of good evidence that selective immunodepression or immune deficiency is a general concomitant of ageing and important in permitting cancer development, it is difficult to see how a decision could be reached as to whether this is a specific biological deficiency or merely part of the general multisystemic functional decline associated with senility. In a practical sense what is important is to identify and measure the defects, assess their relevance and attempt to correct them where possible and appropriate.

Induced Immune Suppression and Cancer

Current medical practice employs many drugs and techniques which depress lymphocyte function *in vitro*. The degree of depression ranges from relatively minor variations in *in vitro* test results associated with agents as commonplace as barbiturates (Trowell, 1958) and nitrous oxide (Bruce and Wingard, 1971) to massive and prolonged alterations after radiotherapy or cytotoxic chemotherapy (Thomas *et al.*, 1971; Ilbery *et al.*, 1971; Glas and Wasserman, 1974; Hersh and Oppenheim, 1967; Hersh *et al.*, 1971; Campbell *et al.*, 1973). The relatively minor reduction of lymphocyte functional efficiency *in vitro* found with many common agents is usually associated with trivial effects *in vivo* and clinically detectable important sequelae are infrequent. By contrast major immunosuppression after radiation or high dose single agent or combined chemotherapy may diminish the body defences against infection to a considerable degree. This is most clearly and significantly demonstrated by the susceptibility of recipients of high-dose chemotherapy to intractable and potentially fatal infections with bacteria and fungi of normally low pathogenicity (so-called opportunistic infections) (Simone *et al.*, 1972; Graham-Pole *et al.*, 1975). It is extremely important to appreciate the difference between even quite severe depression of *in vitro* reactions without clinical effect and the occurrence of a real breach of body defences manifested by opportunistic infection.

Therapeutic immunosuppression is currently employed in two clinical situations. The first is in patients who manifest overactivity or perversion of normal immunological activity or who develop apparently inappropriate immune reactivity against "normal" tissue determinants. The second is in the treatment of recipients of organ allografts where immunosuppression serves to control the entirely predictable host versus graft (allograft) reaction. Both groups of patients provide an interesting opportunity for the epidemiological analysis of the effects of diminished immunological integrity.

There is, in fact, a considerable increase in the incidence of malignancy in immunosuppressed patients relative to non-immunosuppressed individuals of similar age and sex. However, although there is a small increase in the non-allografted, immunosuppressed group (Penn, 1974; Tannenbaum and

Schur, 1974; Roberts and Bell, 1976; Westberg and Swolin, 1976) the overwhelming increase is in the allograft recipients (Penn and Starzl, 1972). It appears that immunosuppression *per se* only slightly increases cancer risk, but that the presence of antigenically foreign material plus immunosuppression is a combination which dramatically favours carcinogenesis. The mechanism of this phenomenon is not known. Schwartz (1972), as noted above, has suggested that the chronic immunological stimulus of even weak graft versus host reaction may be carcinogenic and it is striking that the greatest increase in tumours—the development of lymphomas, affects the tissues most stimulated by antigenic disparity. It has also been suggested that chronic stimulation of the reticuloendothelial system may render it specially sensitive to oncogenic viruses or may activate latent oncogenic viruses. Chronic reticuloendothelial stimulation by malaria has been suggested as a co-factor in the development of Burkitt's lymphoma, a tumour in which there is evidence to suggest that a virus of the herpes group (Epstein-Barr virus) may be aetiologically involved (Burkitt, 1969).

Organ grafting provides another insight into the immunological rejection of foreign cells. Patients have received allografted kidneys which inadvertently contained tumour. In the presence of therapeutically efficient immune suppression the allografted tumour may survive and on occasion has metastasised to organs distant from the kidney. When immune suppression has been discontinued tumour rejection usually occurs but the metastases have *not* always been rejected with the kidney (Penn and Starzl, 1973). This, of course, says nothing about tumour rejection based on tumour-associated antigenic differences. It confirms the existence of transplantation antigens on tumour cells and indicates that large masses of tissue including tumour tissue can be destroyed by immunological mechanisms, if the antigenic "strength" of a graft and its disparity from the recipient are sufficiently high and the recipient adequately immunocompetent. Whether tumour-associated antigens on the highly selected cells of a spontaneous tumour possess sufficient rejection inducing strength or can be modified to produce such rejection inducing characteristics remains a central and crucial, but as yet unanswered question for the tumour immunologist (Klein and Klein, 1977).

A fascinating situation is developing in patients with those few malignancies, such as acute lymphoblastic leukaemia, where advances in chemotherapy now permit previously unattainable lengths of survival. It is not yet known to what degree patients whose lives have been extended in this way are more likely to develop further malignancies of different organs. If this does turn out to be the case, and reports especially recording post-chemotherapy leukaemia are accumulating (Spykens-Smit and Meyler, 1970; Anderson and Videbaeck, 1970; Rosner and Grünwals, 1974; Pariser, 1974), the interpretation of the effect will be complex. It will certainly require consideration of the long term effects of oncogenic agents on the relatively less susceptible organs of the survivors and the possibility of genetic factors dictating susceptibility. From the standpoint of the present discussion, it will also be necessary to consider the extent to which chronic immunosuppression, an inevitable concomitant of the continued administration of all presently available drugs, is important. It will also be important to assess the extent to which environmental carcinogens, including those which induced the original tumour, exert immunosuppression simultaneously with their direct carcinogenicity. In experimental studies both oncogenic viruses and chemical carcinogens have been shown significantly to depress immunity (Peterson et al., 1963; Friedman and Ceglowski, 1968; Rubin, 1964; Stjernswärd, 1969).

Tumour Regression

Total and indefinitely maintained regression of histologically proved malignant disease, although it undoubtedly occurs, is rare. Reports of tumour regression were exhaustively and critically documented by Everson and Cole (1966) who confirmed the rarity of the phenomenon and indicated the meticulous standards of diagnosis and continuing assessment necessary to permit an acceptable claim of a regression. The mechanisms causing such events are probably multiple but are poorly understood. Many regressions have followed inflammation of the tumour site and some have followed periods of pyrexia, the latter observation being the basis of current attempts to treat cancer by hyperthermia. Other factors considered as possibly important in the induction of regression include hormones, metabolic factors, nutrition and removal of the carcinogenic stimulus. There is little direct evidence that the immune system is involved in all or even most regressions, but it is of interest that the tumours most frequently reported as undergoing regression include those in which studies of tumour-related immunity have been most productive. These include adenocarcinoma of the kidney, malignant melanoma, neuroblastoma, choriocarcinoma and Burkitt's lymphoma. We have found tumour-directed cell mediated immunity in all melanoma patients with clinical evidence of (even partial) tumour regression, and this even in patients with advanced disease when the majority would be expected to be non-reactive (Chapter 3). Histological examination of a regressing tumour usually shows destruction of its component cells with an associated lymphocyte and macrophage infiltrate (Fig. 2.1) and after organisation formation of collagenous scar tissue. In some tumours such as neuroblastoma, some events recorded as regression actually represent the maturation of tumour cells into non-malignant forms.

This type of maturation seems confined to the unique conditions of early childhood and is probably merely a fortuitous result of the kinetics of somatic maturation. An understanding of the underlying mechanisms would be of considerable importance and might permit the use of therapeutic induction of maturation as a form of cancer treatment. The low frequency of regression-maturation in other childhood tumours, such as nephroblastoma and hepatoblastoma suggests, however, that the situation is complex.

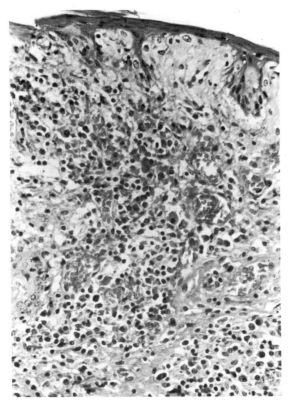

Fig. 2.1. A primary malignant melanoma undergoing spontaneous regression. The tumour is extensively infiltrated by lymphocytes and macrophages. Occasional plasma cells are also present. Haematoxylin and Eosin (× 300).

Total permanent regression of tumours is rare, but partial regression of primary or secondary tumours is rather more common, especially in malignant melanoma (Nathanson, 1976). Bodenham and Lloyd (1963) have described the regression of some cutaneous metastases while other, often adjacent, tumours grew progressively, a situation often seen with "in transit" metastases (Fig. 2.2). It is difficult to see how this could be mediated by systemic specific anti-tumour immunity unless the cells of separate metastases differ in the nature, expression or accessibility of tumour associated antigens.

Partial or total regression may also occur in primary malignant melanomas which may show necrobiosis, focal necrosis, infiltrates of lymphocytes, pigment laden macrophages and foci of intratumoral fibrosis on microscopy (Fig. 2.1) (Smith and Stehlin, 1975; Little, 1972) and grey or grey-pink coloration clinically (Mihm et al., 1973). Metastasis formation may occur prior to or despite such regressive changes, and this interesting local event is not held to have overall prognostic significance. Similar changes are regularly observed in regressing halo naevi (Fig. 2.3), a lesion which has been claimed by some authors to be an early malignant melanoma (Chapter 3).

Another interesting situation is represented by the three to eight per cent of patients who present with melanomatous lymph nodes or visceral metastases without a detectable primary melanoma. Careful examination, with a Wood's lamp if necessary, shows a proportion of such patients to have areas of vitiligo or other pigmentary anomalies and a history of regression of a cutaneous lesion may be elicited from the patient or a relative. Histological examination of the regressed lesion, relatively soon after regression shows few epidermal melanocytes, pigment free in the dermis and in macrophages, lymphocytic infiltration and in some lesions large cells consistent with degenerate melanoma cells. There is no general agreement over the prognostic significance of these events, but I have observed two such cases where there was unusually long survival after excision of tumorous nodes (Cochran et al., 1970).

Regression of a primary tumour is not confined to melanoma, there being for instance, well recorded cases of secondary seminoma in which nothing other than a scar in the testis has been identified. The familial self healing squamous carcinoma of Ferguson-Smith (Ferguson-Smith, 1934) is certainly a special case, but regression of a tumour which closely resembles a primary squamous carcinoma does occur in this condition and there is the added fascination of a genetic link.

Variations in the Rate of Tumour Progression

The majority of cancers are relatively predictable in terms of rate of progression and time from clinical presentation to death. However, some patients survive for periods which are dramatically shorter or longer than expected. This variability is due to many features of host and tumour and the assessment of their relative importance is made more difficult by the need to

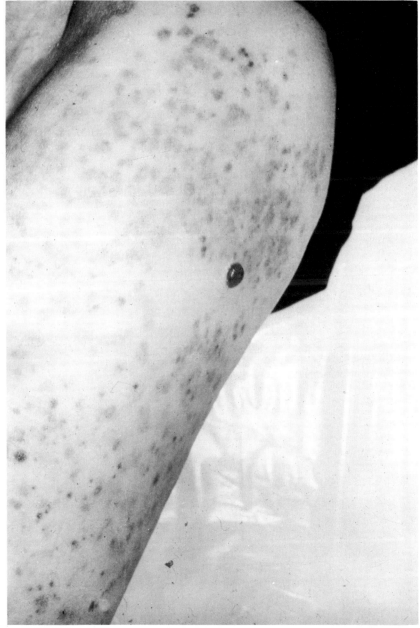

Fig. 2.2. "In transit" metastases of malignant melanoma following excision of a primary tumour and tumorous regional lymph nodes. Some tumours are progressing while others are static or regressing. Photograph by courtesy of Professor T. Gibson.

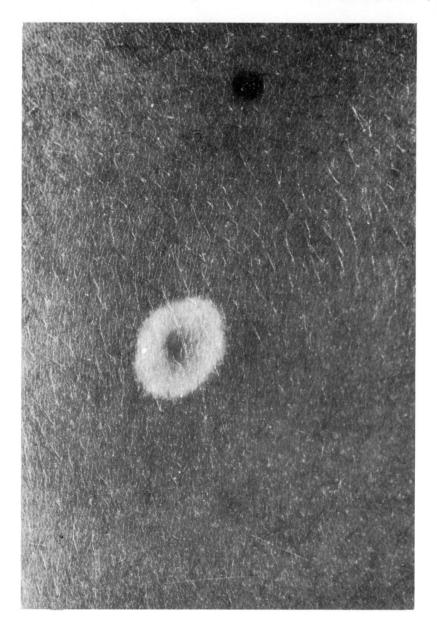

Fig. 2.3. A regressing halo naevus. Note that there is also an adjacent pigmented lesion which is not showing halo formation. Photograph by courtesy of Professor R. M. Mackie.

assess and analyse the effects of different forms of therapy. However, consideration should certainly be given to the role of immunological competence, the effect of chemotherapy, radiotherapy and surgery on immunity, the influence of intercurrent infections or metabolic disease and the significance of endocrine factors.

Cancer patients, especially those on chemotherapy or radiotherapy have a high incidence of infections which, in most cases, appear to have little effect on tumour growth or spread. There are, however, claims that tumour progress has been halted or slowed in some patients following an infection, such as an empyema following surgery for lung cancer (Sensenig et al., 1963). More recent reports of larger series of cases have, however, tended to find empyema an unfavourable event in lung cancer patients (Brohee et al., 1977). It is conceivable that infections might produce a good result if potentially beneficial factors such as pyrexia and the induction of immunogenic neoantigens in infected (tumour) cells by viruses (Steel and Hardy, 1970) outweighed the unfavourable effects of microorganismal toxins and the immunosuppressive effects of corticosteroids (Kelly, 1959) and antibiotics (Zwaveling, 1962).

Tumour and host share the same metabolic environment and requirements and it is therefore inevitable that situations of substrate competition arise from time to time. Decline or functional derangement of major systems such as those controlling urea and electrolyte balance, haemopoiesis or protein synthesis certainly impair the host's capacity to contain malignancy, although the detailed pathways of failure remain to be established.

The relationship of the endocrine system to tumour growth and spread varies widely. Setting aside the relatively hormone dependent cancers of breast and prostate, endocrine factors do, in a minority of patients, seem to influence tumours, usually by increasing their growth, but occasionally by inhibiting it. Few authors would claim malignant melanoma to be hormone-dependent, yet melanoma is rare before sexual maturity, its growth rate may vary during and after pregnancy and occasional patients respond to endocrine therapy. Hormones may act directly on tumour cells, but there is increasing interest in interactions between the endocrine and immunological systems, which have to be considered in assessing endocrine effects. For example, lung tumours which secrete "inappropriate" adrenocorticotrophin-like material have a worse prognosis than histologically similar tumours which do not produce hormones and this difference may be due in part to the immunosuppressive effect of the hormones produced by the stimulated adrenal cortex and in part to a direct effect of such hormones on the tumour cells. Another potentially important area which is little understood is the relationship between apparently psychological factors such as the patient's attitude to and knowledge of the significance of his disease and emotional trauma such as bereavement which may immediately precede the appearance of clinically detectable metastatic disease. Links between the central nervous system and the endocrine system certainly exist and may be crucial in triggering alterations in the host-tumour relationship.

Tumour Latency and Dormancy

Some patients with histologically proved malignancy remain clinically tumour free for many years after ostensibly successful tumour surgery and yet after this time develop metastases histologically and functionally identical to the primary. The best example of this known to the author is a woman with malignant melanoma who survived twenty three years (and two professors of pathology) before developing and dying from visceral metastases. The implication is that small numbers of residual tumour cells lie dormant for many years only to re-emerge when the balance of the host-tumour relationship alters. There is no proof that this explanation is correct and it is difficult to see how such proof could be obtained. The long latent period may merely reflect the time necessary for a small number of slow growing tumour cells to develop to a clinically detectable level, but the growth rate of such tumours after detection makes this unlikely. We do not know that immunological factors are important in containing latent tumour cells and maintaining their dormancy but it seems a role for which the immune system is well suited.

Histological Observations

A proportion of tumours are attended by an infiltrate of lymphocytes, plasma cells and macrophages which may lie around the tumour periphery (Fig. 2.4) or less commonly be dispersed through it (Fig. 2.5). In some tumours, especially seminoma of testis, the infiltrate may be associated with granulomatous lesions (Fig. 2.6). These are the histological features of an immunological reaction of the type we see in organ-specific autoimmune disease such as Hashimoto's thyroiditis (Fig. 2.7). In the absence of a source of exogenous antigens or massive tumour cell necrosis it is reasonable to consider that such reactions in and around tumours are a response to tumour neoantigens. If this is true patients with tumours showing a reaction might be expected to have a better than average prognosis. This appears to be true in patients with breast carcinoma (Berg, 1959), gastric carcinoma (Black and Speer, 1958), Hodgkin's disease (Lukes, 1964) and neuroblastoma (Martin and Beckwith, 1968) but the situation is less clear with other tumours. In malignant melanoma, with the exception of Thompson (1972) most authors have not reported a better survival for patients with lymphoid-cell associated

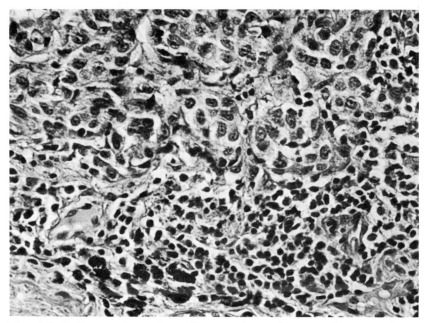

Fig. 2.4. Infiltrate of reactive cells around a primary malignant melanoma. Haematoxylin and Eosin (× 400).

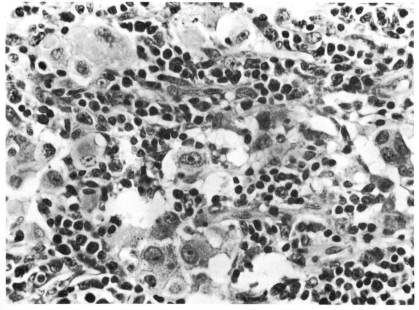

Fig. 2.5. Malignant melanoma infiltrated by reactive cells. Haematoxylin and Eosin (× 600).

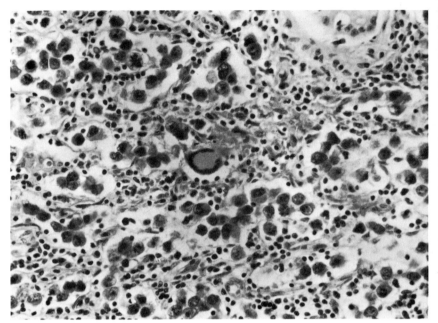

Fig. 2.6. Seminoma infiltrated by reactive cells and showing a granuloma. Haematoxylin and Eosin (× 350).

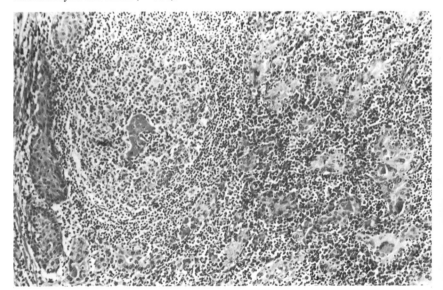

Fig. 2.7. Cellular infiltrate in autoimmune thyroiditis. Note germinal follicle containing a focus of amyloid. (Hashimoto's disease.) Haematoxylin and Eosin (× 125).

tumours. In a study of this problem (Cochran, 1969) I found that local recurrences were significantly less frequent in those individuals with cellular aggregation around their tumours, which may be interpreted as suggesting a *locally* effective defensive role for the involved cells.

The extent of cellular infiltration tends to decrease as the cancer advances and metastasises (Allen and Spitz, 1953; Cochran, 1969). Examination of an invasive malignant melanoma arising in an area of lentigo maligna usually shows a dense population of lymphoid cells beneath the lentigous area while the vertically invasive nodule is often attended by a scanty or patchy infiltrate or no infiltrate at all (Fig. 2.8). Metastatic tumours are relatively seldom accompanied by lymphocytic infiltrates, even though the primary was heavily infiltrated by such cells. These differences are capable of interpretation in several ways. It seems probable that tumour cell characteristics alter between the preinvasive or early invasive phase and the fully developed vertically invasive phase and between primary and secondary deposits. These changes may be part of the spontaneous evolution of the tumour or may be the result of selective growth and multiplication in the face of environmental pressures; such as an anti-tumour immune response and varying hormonal milieu. The changes which we see in evolving tumours are generally in the direction of producing cells which are less and less readily identifiable as antigenically foreign. Such changes may be mediated by antigen deletion, antigen modulation or the introduction or expansion of a system of antigen masking. The observed effects could also indicate the development of specific tolerance. The continued presence of lymphocytic aggregates to "premalignant areas" around invasive melanomas and the variable aggrega- tion of lymphoid cells around adjacent but cytologically different areas of tumour cells within a primary melanoma (Clark et al, 1976) (Fig. 4.3) "make it unlikely that tolerance is important in this situation".

Ultrastructural and experimental studies of peritumoral cells have as yet added little to our understanding of their function. Carr and Underwood (1974), in an electron-microscopic study of these cells found that they appeared to be undergoing "instruction" rather than functioning as effector (killer) cells. Cesarini and Roubin (1975) have cast doubt on the conventional light micro- scopic interpretation of the nature of these cells, claiming that, on the basis of ultrastructure, the majority of them are members of the monocyte series. The technical difficulty of obtaining peritumoral "lymphocytes" in numbers and condition suitable for experimental assessment has severely limited such studies. As a result of this limitation most studies of the immunological activity of these cells have been rather negative. This topic is reviewed in detail in Chapter 3. In a study of peripheral leucocytes from patients with primary melanomas we found no difference in reaction frequency between those from patients with tumours showing heavy "lymphocytic" aggregation

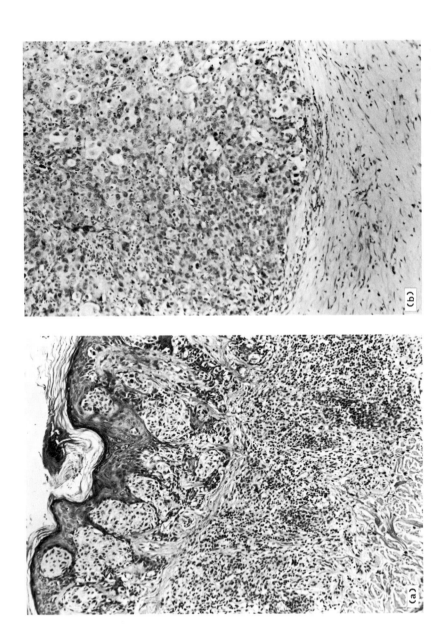

Fig. 2.8. Malignant melanoma. The reactive cellular infiltrate is maximum beneath the area of melanoma-*in-situ* (Figure a) and reduced in the area below the invasive component (Figure b). Haematoxylin and Eosin (a × 150; b × 250).

and those whose tumours showed no such aggregation (Mackie *et al.*, 1973).

It has also been claimed that histological examination of excised non-tumorous lymph nodes (excision of such nodes is however, considered a heinous crime by some authorities!) can give some indication of prognosis. Detectable patterns such as sinus histiocytosis, degenerative sinus histiocytosis and sarcoid-like granulomas are certainly identifiable and may indeed have prognostic significance. Black (1973) points out that the areas of node involved favour the activation of cell-mediated, rather than humoral immunity. It is, of course in the draining lymph nodes that early and possibly very significant contact between tumour antigens and immunocytes would be expected to occur. However, prognostication on this basis is limited by the need to excise nodes which may have an important defensive activity and by the fact that different nodes, even those situated closely together may show very different patterns.

Other histological features which might be interpreted as evidence of a host response are the signs of regression discussed above, the desmoplastic reaction and capsule formation. If desmoplasia is a manifestation of a host response, there is little evidence that it is effective; patients with scirrhous breast carcinomas having no apparent survival advantage over women with encephaloid tumours. The traditional view that peritumoral fibrosis represents a host reaction has to be reconsidered in view of studies by Al-Adnani *et al.* (1975) in which evidence was presented that some breast cancer cells possess the enzymes needed for collagen synthesis. The desmoplastic "reaction" may require reassignment as an index of "inappropriate" functional activity of breast cancer cells.

Cancer in Families

In addition to truly hereditary cancer predispositions such as those involved in retinoblastoma, xeroderma pigmentosum, and polyposis coli, there is evidence that blood relatives of patients with a particular type of malignancy have an increased risk of developing the same type of malignancy. Reasonably convincing evidence of this phenomenon exists in the case of breast cancer in women, the leukaemias, colo-rectal cancer and lung cancer (for a review of this topic see Heston, 1976). While it is not yet possible to exclude absolutely carcinogenic agents resulting from common environmental factors in these families the evidence is that, in most situations of this type, the family members possess some heritable anomaly which renders them susceptible to cancer of the appropriate type, there being no general increase in other kinds of cancer. It has recently been shown that the occurrence, degree and quality of an immune response to any given antigen is heritable and depends on "immune responsiveness" (Ir) genes, some of which are closely associated with histocompatibility loci (McDevitt and Benacerraf, 1969). Muhlbock and Dux (1974) have shown that an Ir gene linked to the H-2 (histocompatibility) locus influences the development of breast tumours in mice exposed to the mammary tumour virus. Work on Ir genes, to date has involved highly specific antigens, but it will certainly be crucial to ascertain whether familial cancer susceptibility is due, at least in part, to genetically determined inadequacy of Ir genes. The study of associations between particular HL-A types and disease may provide some indirect information on this point. Associations between non-malignant disease and particular HL-A types have been reported, such as a high frequency of HL-A27 in ankylosing spondylitis. Studies of HL-A type in patients with malignant disease have been disappointingly inconclusive, but studies of haplotype are more promising. There is, for instance, said to be an increase of haplotype W30-HL-A12 in malignant melanoma and of HL-A 9-5 in lymphomas. These studies are highly complicated but seem likely to yield exciting data in the next decade.

Multiple Primary Tumours

The simultaneous occurrence of more than one malignancy is rare, but the sequential development of different malignancies is not uncommon (Moertel, 1966). As patients who have had one cancer have an increased likelihood of developing a second, increased success in treating malignancy will probably lead to more patients developing multiple malignancies. The mechanisms involved are not clear. We may be seeing the effect of further cumulated carcinogenic exposure or the late response of relatively less carcinogen-sensitive organs. It is also possible that the affected individuals are immuno-suppressed and thus lack the protection of an intact surveillance mechanism. Immunosuppressive factors to be considered include the carcinogens, ageing (multiple cancers occur maximally in the elderly—Serrou et al., 1974), treatments applied to the initial malignancy, including radiotherapy, and chemotherapy and residual debilitation from the initial malignancy.

Circulating Tumour Cells

A curious recurring observation is that tumour cells are identifiable in the blood of cancer patients even at an early stage and long before metastases develop (Engell, 1955; Moore and Sandberg, 1957; Madden and Karpas, 1967). Quantification of these cells indicates that the overwhelming majority do not establish progressively growing metastases. This is certainly convincing evidence that highly efficient mechanisms for tumour cell destruction and containment do exist, although their nature remains a matter of speculation. Even the clinical significance of this observation is debatable, Watne *et al.* (1960) claimed it to presage an unfavourable outcome, a view however not shared by others (Engell, 1959; Roberts *et al.*, 1961; Romsdahl *et al.*, 1965).

Treatment Responses

There are well documented reports of cancer patients whose disease has regressed or failed to progress despite their having received treatment which, by conventional standards, was less than adequate. Examples are patients with Burkitt's lymphoma (Burkitt *et al.*, 1969) or choriocarcinoma whose tumours have responded to a dose of chemotherapy which would not conventionally be expected to be active and patients whose metastases have regressed after excision or diathermy or cryotherapy of a primary tumour. The standard, plausible if unproven, explanation of these events is that the therapy initiates regressive changes in the tumours which are then completed by physiological mechanisms.

Trophoblastic Malignancies

These are unique as tumours of one individual (the foetus) which grow and metastasise in and may lead to the death of another (the mother). The tumour cells derive genetic material from both mother and father and are thus half allogeneic to the mother and are therefore in essence an allograft. Choriocarcinoma, the most malignant trophoblastic neoplasm, undergoes spontaneous regression relatively frequently and responds well to chemotherapy, in some cases at relatively low dose. The significance of this latter finding is discussed above. Evidence of the importance of immunological aspects of choriocarcinoma, comes from studies where immunotherapy of the tumour has achieved some success—using either paternal leucocytes (Cinader *et al.*, 1961) or xeno-antisera raised against paternal spermatozoa (Jakoubkova *et al.*, 1965). Rejection of paternal skin grafts may be slow and may not be associated with production of the expected agglutinins to the donor's leucocytes (Robinson *et al.*, 1963).

Other Observations

There are numerous bizarre clinical phenomena associated with malignant disease such as acanthosis nigricans, dermatomyositis, erythema annulare centrifugum, haemolytic anaemias, and neuromyopathies (for review see Azzopardi, 1966). The mechanisms associated with these conditions are not totally understood but in some at least immunological factors are important, probably largely dependent upon cross reactions between structurally similar antigens on tumour cells and normal tissues.

Summary

There are numerous clinical and pathological observations which support the existence of host factors which act to minimise the chance of tumour development and which may also impede the progress of established tumours. Such observations indicate those situations which are most likely to be of interest to the investigator. In a few instances immunological factors are involved; in the majority of cases the nature of the complicated mechanisms remains quite unknown.

References

Al-Adnani, M. S. and McGee, J. O. (1975). *Brit. J. Cancer* **31**, 653.
Allen, A. C. and Spitz, S. (1953). *Cancer* **6**, 1-45.
Anderson, E. and Videbaek, A. (1970). *Scand. J. Haematol.* **7**, 201-207.
Azzopardi, J. G. (1966). *In* "Recent Advances in Pathology" (C. V. Harrison, Ed.) 8th Edition, 98-184. Churchill, London.
Berg, J. W. (1959). *Cancer* **12**, 714-740.
Black, M. M., Opler, S. R. and Speer, F. D. (1954). *Surg. Gynec. Obstet.* **98**, 725-734.
Black, M. M. and Speer, F. D. (1958). *Surg. Gynec. Obstet.* **106**, 163-175.
Black, M. M. (1973). *In* "Immunological Parameters of host-tumor relationships" (D. Weiss, Ed.) Vol. II, 80-95. Academic Press, New York and London.
Bodenham, D. C. and Lloyd, O. C. (1963). *Postgrad. med. J.* **39**, 278-279.
Brohee, D., Vanderhoeft, P. and Smets, P. (1977). *Europ. J. Cancer.* **13**, 1429.
Bruce, D. L. and Wingard, D. W. (1971). *Anesthesiology* **34**, 271-282.
Burkitt, D. P. (1969). *J. nat. Cancer Inst.* **42**, 19-28.
Burnet, F. M. (1967). *Lancet* **1**, 1171-1174.
Burnet, F. M. (1970). *Progr. Exptl. Tumor. Res.* **13**, 1-27.
Campbell, A. C., Hersey, P., MacLennan, I. C. M., Kay, H. E. M., Pike, M. C. and MRC Working Party on Leukaemia in Childhood (1973). *Brit. med. J.* **2**, 385-388.
Cantor, H., Asofsky, R. and Talal, N. (1970). *J. exp. Med.* **131**, 223-234.
Carr, I. and Underwood, J. C. E. (1974). *Int. Rev. Cytol.* **37**, 329-347.
Cesarini, J.-P. and Roubin, R. (1975). *Behring Inst. Mitt.* **56**, 65-73.
Cinader, B., Haley, M. A., Rider, W. D., Warwick, D. H. (1961). *Canad. med. Ass. J.* **84**, 306-000.
Clark, W. H., Ainsworth, A. M., Bernardino, E. A., Yang, C.-H., Mihm, M. C. and Reed, R. J. (1975). *Sem. in Oncol.* **2**, 83-103.
Cochran, A. J. (1969). *J. Pathol.* **97**, 459-468.
Cochran, A. J., Diehl, V. and Stjernswärd, J. (1970). *Rev. Europ. Etudes Clin. et Biol.* **15**, 969-972.
Engell, H. C. (1955). *Acta chir. Scand. Suppl.* **201**, 1-70.

Engell, H. C. (1959). *Ann. Surg.* **149**, 457-461.
Epstein, W. L., Fudenberg, H. H., Reed, W. B., Boder, E. and Sedgwick, R. P. (1966). *Int. Arch. Allergy* **30**, 15-29.
Everson, T. C. and Cole, W. H. (1966). Spontaneous Regression of Cancer. Saunders, Philadelphia.
Ferguson-Smith, J. (1934). *Brit. J. Derm.* **46**, 267-272.
Friedman, H. and Ceglowski, W. S. (1968). *Nature* **218**, 1232-1234.
Gatti, R. A. and Good, R. A. (1971). *Cancer* **28**, 89-98.
Glas, U. and Wasserman, J. (1974). *Acta Radiol. (Ther.)* **13**, 185-200.
Govaerts, A. (1976). *In* "Clinical Tumour Immunology" (J. Wybran and M. Staquet, Eds.) 107-114. Pergamon Press, Oxford.
Graham-Pole, J., Willoughby, M. L. N., Aitken, S. and Ferguson, A. (1975). *Brit. med. J.* **2**, 467-470.
Hallgren, H. M. and Wood, N. E. (1972). *Fed. Proc.* **31**, 649-655.
Hersh, E. M. and Oppenheim, J. J. (1967). *Cancer Res.* **27**, 98-105.
Hersh, E. M., Whitecar, J. P., McCredie, K. B., Bodey, G. P., Freireich, E. J. (1971). *New Engl. J. Med.* **285**, 1211-1216.
Heston, W. E. (1976). *In* "Advances in Cancer Research" (G. Klein and S. Weinhouse, Eds.) Vol. 23, 1-22. Academic Press, New York and London.
Huber, J. (1968). *In* "Immunological Deficiency Diseases in Man". Birth Defects Original Article Series, No. 4, New York.
Humphreys, S. R., Glynn, J. P., Chirigos, M. A. and Goldin, A. (1962). *J. Nat. Cancer Inst.* **28**, 1053-1063.
Ilbery, P. L. T., Rickinson, A. B. and Thrum, C. E. (1971). *Brit. J. Radiol.* **44**, 834-840.
Jakoubkova, J., Koldovsky, P., Bek, V., Majsky, A., Schneid, V. and Vopotova, M. (1965). *Neoplasma* **12**, 131-135.
Kelly, M. (1959). *Acta rheum. Scand.* **5**, 286-290.
Kishimoto, S., Tsuyuguchi, I. and Yamamura, Y. (1969). *Clin. exp. Immunol.* **5**, 525-530.
Kishimoto, S., Shigemoto, S. and Hayamura, Y. (1974). *Transplant* **15**, 455-459.
Klein, G. and Klein, E. (1977). *Transplant Proc.* **9**, 1095.
Lardye, G. J. (1973). *Lancet* **1**, 641-643.
Little, J. H. (1972). *In* "Melanoma and Skin Cancer" (McCarthy, W. H. Ed.) Government Printer, Sydney.
Lukes, R. J. (1964). *J. Amer. med. Ass.* **190**, 914-915.
Mackie, R. M., Spilg, W. G. S., Thomas, C. E., Cameron-Mowat, D. E., Grant, R. M. and Cochran, A. J. (1973). *Rev. Inst. Pasteur de Lyon* **6**, 281-290.
Madden, R. E. and Karpas, C. M. (1967). *Arch. Surg.* **94**, 307-312.
Martin, R. F. and Beckwith, J. B. (1968). *J. Ped. Surg.* **3**, 106-110.
Mihm, M. C., Fitzpatrick, T. B. and Lane-Brown, M. M. *et al.* (1973). *New Engl. J. Med.* **289**, 989-995.
Moertel, C. G. (1966). "Multiple Primary Malignant Neoplasms". Springer, Heidelberg.
Moore, G. E., Sandberg, A. and Schubarg, J. R. (1954). *Ann. Surg.* **146**, 580-587.
Morton, J. L. and Siegel, B. V. (1968). *J. Reticuloendoth. Soc.* **6**, 78-93.
Muhlbock, O. and Dux, A. (1974). *J. nat. Cancer Inst.* **53**, 993-996.
McDevitt, H. D. and Benacerraf, B. (1969). *Advan. Immunol.* **11**, 31-50.
McKay, I. R. (1972). *Gerontologia (Basel)* **18**, 285-304.
Nathanson, L. (1976). *Nat. Cancer Inst. Monogr.* **44**, 67-76.

Pariser, S. (1974). *N. Y. State J. Med.* **74**, 2016-2023.
Penn, I. and Starzl, T. E. (1972). *Transplant* **14**, 407-417.
Penn, I. and Starzl, T. E. (1973). *Transplant Proc.* **5**, 943-947.
Penn, I. (1974). *Cancer* **34**, 858-866.
Peterson, R. D. A., Hendrickson, R. and Good, R. A. (1963). *Proc. Soc. exp. Biol. Med.* **114**, 517-520.
Potter, C. W., Hoskins, J. M. and Oxford, J. S. (1969). *Arch. Gesante Virus forsch.* **27**, 73-86.
Prehn, R. T. (1970). *In* "Immune Surveillance" (R. T. Smith and M. Landy, Eds.) Academic Press, New York and London.
Prehn, R. T. (1971). *J. Reticuloendothel. Soc.* **10**, 1-16.
Prehn, R. T. and Lappé, M. A. (1971). *Transplant Rev.* **7**, 26-40.
Prehn, R. T. (1972). *Science* **176**, 170-171.
Roberts, S. S., Jonasson, O., Long, L., McGrath, R., McGrew, E. A. and Cole, W. H. (1961). *Ann. Surg.* **154**, 362-371.
Roberts, M. M. and Bell, R. (1976). *Lancet* **2**, 768-770.
Robinson, E., Schulman, J., Ben-Hur, N., Zuckerman, H. and Neuman, Z. (1963). *Lancet* **1**, 300-302.
Rodey, G. E., Good, R. A. and Yunis, E. J. (1971). *Clin. exp. Immunol.* **9**, 305-311.
Romsdahl, M. M., Valaitis, J., McGrath, R. G. and McGrew, E. A. (1965). *J. Amer. med. Ass.* **193**, 1087-1090.
Rosner, F. and Grünwald, H. (1974). *Amer. J. Med.* **57**, 927-939.
Rowley, M. J. and McKay, I. R. (1969). *Clin. exp. Immunol.* **15**, 407-418.
Rubin, B. A. (1964). *Progr. exp. Tumour Res.* **5**, 217-233.
Schwartz, R. B. (1972). *Lancet* **1**, 1266-1269.
Sensenig, D. M., Rossi, N. P. and Ehrenhaft, J. L. (1963). *Surg. Gynec. Obstet.* **116**, 279-284.
Serrou, B., Dubois, J. B. and Romieu, C. (1974). *Nouv. Presse med.* **3**, 1369-1371.
Simone, J. V., Holland, E. and Johnson, W. (1972). *Blood* **39**, 759-770.
Smith, J. S. and Stehlin, J. S. (1965). *Cancer* **18**, 1399-1415.
Spykens-Smit, C. G. and Meyler, L. (1970). *Lancet* **2**, 671-672.
Steel, C. M. and Hardy, D. A. (1970). *Lancet* **1**, 1322-1323.
Stjernswärd, J. (1966). *J. Nat. Cancer Inst.* **37**, 505-512.
Stjernswärd, J. (1969). *Antibiotica Chemotherap.* **15**, 213-218.
Stutman, O., Yunis, E. J. and Good, R. A. (1968). *Proc. Soc. exp. Biol. Med.* **127**, 1204.
Tannenbaum, H. and Schur, P. H. (1974). *Arthritis Rheum.* **17**, 15-18.
Thomas, L. (1959). *In* "Cellular and Humoral aspects of the hypersensitivity state" (Lawrence, H. S. Ed.) 529. Hoeber, New York.
Thomas, J. M., Coy, P., Lewis, H. S. and Yuen, A. (1971). *Cancer* **27**, 1046-1050.
Thompson, P. (1972). *In* "Proceedings of VIIIth International Pigment Cell Conference". Australian Government Printer, Sydney, 100 (Abstract).
Trowell, O. A. (1958). *Biochem. Pharmacol.* **1**, 288-295.
Walford, R. L. (1969). "The Immunologic Theory of Ageing". Munksgaard, Copenhagen.
Walford, R. L. (1974). *Fed. Proc.* **33**, 2020-2027.
Watne, A. L., Roberts, S. S., McGrew, E. A. and Cole, W. H. (1960). *Acta Un. Int. Cancer* **16**, 790-799.
Weber, J. C. and Schlaegel, T. F. (1969). *Amer. J. Ophthal.* **67**, 732-737.
Westberg, N. G. and Swolin, B. (1976). *Acta med. Scand.* **199**, 373-377.

Whittingham, S. J., Irwin, J. and McKay, I. R. (1969). *Aust. Ann. Med.* **18,** 130-134.
Wigzell, H. and Stjernswärd, J. (1966). *J. Nat. Cancer Inst.* **37,** 513-517.
Zwaveling, A. (1962). *Cancer* **15,** 790-796.

3

Immunological Responses Against Tumour Cells

If human tumours bear (surface) antigens which differ from those on normal cells they should evoke detectable immune responses which could, under optimal conditions, induce regression or prevent or retard metastasis formation. Even if such responses do not inhibit tumour progression, detection and quantification of anti-tumour antibodies and specifically sensitised lymphoid cells may be of value in diagnosis, staging, and monitoring for the development of metastases. It may also be useful to detect and monitor the effects of reactions between tumour antigens and anti-tumour antibodies by measuring immune complexes, assessing the ratio of antigen to antibody in such complexes and measuring complement activation.

Tumour Grafts

Tumour inhibition, either spontaneous or, after immunisation of groups of carcinogen or tumour transplant challenged animals is the strongest available evidence of an effector role for immunity in tumour control.

In man, graft studies have been limited by ethical considerations, but those which have been undertaken have produced information of considerable interest. Patients have had portions of their own tumours (autografts) reimplanted (Grace, 1964; Nadler and Moore, 1965; McLellan, 1969) and a surprisingly small number of such implants have grown. Southam (1965) reported that tumour autograft acceptance correlated with inoculum size, with the acceptance of tumour allografts, with skin reactivity to tuberculoprotein and DNCB and with macrophage function. Mixing blood leucocytes with tumour cells increases the number of cells necessary for outgrowth of a tumour graft, indicating that some component of the leucocytes can inhibit tumour cells. Tumour cells have also been transferred from one individual to another (allografts). When the recipients are normal or have non-malignant diseases rejection of tumour allografts is virtually always normal (Levin *et al.*, 1964). However immunosuppressed individuals without malignant disease may permit local growth of allogeneic tumour cells and rarely metastases develop and cause death (Scanlon *et al.*, 1965).

Most cancer patients, even those with metastases, reject tumour allografts (Arata *et al.*, 1969) but rejection is slow in a proportion. It is reasonably acceptable to allograft tumour cells between cancer patients to raise antibodies or sensitised lymphocytes or transfer factor, but the recipient may at the same time receive genome material of oncogenic or other pathogenic viruses. While such transfer is not a short term problem, achievement of lengthy survival might permit the induction and development of a second malignancy.

Antibodies Directed Against Tumour Cells

Antibodies may be sought free in plasma or other body fluids or attached to their natural substrate, the tumour cells.

FREE CIRCULATING ANTIBODIES

A considerable increase in circulating antibodies may be associated with a rise in plasma immunoglobulins (Ig) detectable by a simple radial immuno-diffusion technique (Mancini *et al.*, 1965). Whether an increase in total Ig is present or not it is mandatory to demonstrate that any alteration in the Ig content of serum is due to the development or expansion of antibody Ig with specificity for tumour-associated antigens. Many techniques exist for the identification of antibodies and virtually all have been used to search for anti-tumour antibodies. They vary widely in technical difficulty and sensitivity, which factors have dictated the techniques most widely employed. Some of the more commonly employed techniques are listed in Table 3.1. The existence of multiple techniques indicates the lack of an ideal test combining technical simplicity and absolute discriminatory capacity.

A detailed technical analysis is beyond the scope of this monograph and the interested reader is referred to recent reviews (Cochran, 1978; Baldwin and Embleton, 1976). The following merely highlights major technical problems.

Immunofluorescence techniques

Indirect tests with serum have been widely used to detect antibodies to cytoplasmic antigens in dead cells and membrane antigens on living cells.

Table 3.1.

Techniques for the detection of tumour-directed antibodies in body fluids

1. Detection of Ig *on* or *in* tumour cells by labelled anti-Ig sera. *Immunofluorescence and immunoperoxidase techniques* (Klein *et al.*, 1966; Kuhlmann and Miller, 1971).

2. Adherence of erythrocytes to tumour cells in the presence of antibody and complement, *immune adherence* (Nishioka, 1963).

3. Antibody mediated complement dependent tumour cell lysis, *serum cytotoxicity* (Slettenmark and Klein, 1962).

4. Inhibition of tumour cell growth and replication *in vitro, serum cytostasis* (Hellström and Sjogren, 1965).

5. Inhibition of tumour cell movement *in vitro, migration inhibition* (Cochran, 1971).

6. Cross-binding of human antibody-coated sheep erythrocytes by anti-human Ig to antibody-coated tumour cells, *mixed haemadsorption* (Fagraeus and Epsmark, 1961).

7. Killing of antibody-coated tumour cells by non-sensitised mononuclear (K) cells, *antibody dependent cell-mediated* cytotoxicity (McLennan *et al.*, 1969).

8. Precipitation of interacting tumour antigens and antibodies, *precipitation* (Winters and Morton, 1973).

9. Complement fixation during antigen-antibody reactions, *complement fixation* (Odili and Taylor, 1971).

Relative technical simplicity is associated with problems of interpretation and choice of target cells. Tumour imprints and cytocentrifuge preparations although cytologically heterogeneous, are easier to interpret than frozen sections, but identification of tumour cells remains a problem. Cells coated with Ig *in vivo* present interpretational problems, resolvable by direct tests with anti-Ig sera. Monolayer or suspension cultures provide alternative target cells but are not always available for autologous tests and are sometimes difficult to identify as tumorous. They may undergo antigenic alteration during culture; loss of HL-A antigens (Sasportes *et al.*, 1971); re-expression of embryonal antigens (Stonehill and Bendich, 1970), acquisition of tissue-specific antigens (Herschman and Lerner, 1973) and acquisition of antigens from medium additives such as fetal calf serum (Irie *et al.*, 1974; Sulit *et al.*, 1976).

Problems of subjectivity of assessment may be answered by automated analysis employing photometric apparatus (Goldman, 1968; Nairn *et al.*, 1969) or comparator microscopy (Haskell and Richmond, 1973). As this technology remains imperfect and the equipment expensive visual assessment is likely to remain standard for some time.

Immune adherence techniques

There has recently been a renewal of interest in this approach, associated with minor modifications (deVries *et al.*, 1975; Macher *et al.*, 1975) of the original methods (Nelson, 1953; Nishioka, 1963a and b). Problems in providing good reactive target cells may be overcome by formalin fixation (Macher *et al.*, 1975; Cochran *et al.*, 1976) but visual rosette counting remains tedious and should be automated. Sensitivity is rather less than that of immunofluorescence techniques.

Antibody related cytotoxicity and cytostasis

These theoretically simple tests (Slettenmark and Klein, 1962; Old *et al.*, 1963) are limited by variations in tumour cell sensitivity to the attentions of antibody, variable rates of isotope uptake and subsequent release by tumour cells and the fact that not all antibodies are cytotoxic. If short term complement dependent cytotoxicity studies are not satisfactory longer term examination of antibody mediated cell killing or growth inhibition are possible (Hellström and Hellström, 1970) or cell mediated cytotoxicity of antibody primed target cells may be assessed (McLennan, 1976).

Tumour cell migration

Given a motile population of tumour cells (usually lymphomas) (Cochran, 1971; Cochran *et al.*, 1973) antibodies to transplantation antigens and tumour associated antigens may be identified by their ability to inhibit the escape of tumour cells from capillary tubes (Cochran *et al.*, 1972; Currie and Sime, 1973). This is a very sensitive technique, limited only by the need for a motile indicator cell population.

Other techniques employed with some success include precipitation assays, complement fixation and mixed haemadsorption (Table 3.1).

RESULTS OF STUDIES OF CIRCULATING ANTIBODIES

Incidence in cancer and control populations

Circulating antibodies with relative specificity for appropriate tumour cells have been found in most cancer populations studied (Table 3.2). They are

Table 3.2.

Some reports of circulating tumour-directed antibodies describing a higher incidence
in cancer patients than control donors

Tumour	Technique[a]	Reference
Bladder cancer	CDC	Bubenik et al. (1970) Int. J. Cancer 5, 39
Breast cancer	IF	Edynak et al. (1972) J. nat. Cancer Inst. 48, 1137
Breast cancer	Inhibition labelled antibodies	Gorsky et al. (1976) Proc. nat. Acad. Sci. 73, 2101
Burkitt's lymphoma	CDC	Osunkoya (1967) Brit. J. Cancer 21, 302
Burkitt's lymphoma	IF	Henle et al. (1969) J. nat. Cancer Inst. 43, 1147
Carcinoma cervix	Anticomplement IF	Ito et al. (1976) Int. J. Cancer 18, 557
Colon cancer	IF, CDC	Nairn et al. (1971) Brit. med. J. 4, 706
Hodgkin's disease	IF	Johansson et al. (1970) Int. J. Cancer 6, 450
Leukaemia	IA	Doré et al. (1967) Lancet 2, 1396.
Leukaemia	CDC	Leventhal et al. (1972) Cancer Res. 32, 1820
Melanoma	IF	Morton and Malmgren (1968) Science 162, 1279
Melanoma	IF, CDC	Lewis et al. (1969) Brit. med. J. 3, 547
Melanoma: sarcoma	IF, CF	Morton et al. (1971) Progr. exp. Tumor Res. 14, 25
Melanoma	IF	Whitehead (1973) Brit. J. Cancer 28, 525
Melanoma	IA	Macher et al. (1975) Behring Inst. Mitt. 56, 86
Melanoma	MHA	Carey et al. (1976) Proc. nat. Acad. Sci. 73, 3278
Nasopharyngeal cancer	IF	deSchryver et al. (1970) Clin. exp. Immunol. 7, 161
Sarcomas	IF	Moore et al. (1973) Int. J. Cancer 12, 428
Sarcomas	Precipitation	Winters and Morton (1973) See reference list
Skin cancer	IF, CDC	Nairn et al. (1971) Brit. med. J. 4, 701
Various	IA	Irie et al. (1974) Science 186, 454

[a]IF = immunofluorescence, CDC = complement dependent antibody mediated cytotoxicity,
P = precipitation, MHA = mixed haemadsorption, CF = complement fixation, IA = immune
adherence.

not, however, confined to cancer patients and are found in (usually) around 20% of control individuals. Although possibly due to technical artefact this raises questions concerning the specificity of these antibodies. The simplest concept is of neo-antigens unique to carcinogen-influenced cells, including tumour cells. Antibodies to such antigens could occur in individuals with growing or regressing tumours and those who had had a tumour reduced by treatment. They might also occur in clinically normal people after abortive carcinogen contact or where tumour had regressed subclinically. Alternatively, apparently tumour-specific antigens may exist on normal adult cells at low concentrations or in a masked state, increased frequency or exposure on tumour cells perhaps rendering them immunogenic. Mechanisms other than carcinogenesis may enhance the immunogenicity of such antigens in some tumour free individuals inducing tumour cross-reactive antibodies. Oncofoetal (OF) antigens such as alpha-fetoprotein and carcinoembryonic antigen exist at high concentration on embryo and tumour cells and are absent or infrequent on normal adult cells (see Chapter 4). Reports of antibodies to *known* OF antigens are infrequent but some apparently tumour-antigen directed antibodies may in fact be specific for *unidentified* OF antigens.

Reaction of cancer sera with allogeneic tumours of similar histogenesis (see below) raises the possibility that the antigens detected are organ-specific or transplantation antigens rather than tumour-specific. Organ-specificity is discounted to some extent by the infrequency of reactions against normal tissues, although the critical difference may again be quantitative rather than qualitative. On the basis of the similar frequency of autologous and allogeneic reactions and of the differing reaction frequencies in comparable (age, sex, parity, transfusion history) cancer and control groups it is unlikely that the antibodies detected are against major transplantation antigens. The situation in relation to minor antigens is less clear and antibodies to antigens similar to blood group antigens may simulate anti-tumour antibodies (Bloom *et al.*, 1973).

Recent reports suggest increased autoantibodies against smooth muscle, nuc proteins and bile canaliculi in cancer sera (Ablin and Soanes, 1971; Burnham, 1972; Moore and Hughes, 1973; Whitehouse, 1973) perhaps due to carcinogen induced alteration of antigens or tumour necrosis. Necrosis certainly can induce autoantibodies (Ehrenfeld *et al.*, 1961; Quismorio *et al.*, 1971; Johnsonn *et al.*, 1968). This type of antibody must be sought although the frequency of autoantibodies varies from tumour to tumour and some studies have not found them increased in cancer patients (Nairn *et al.*, 1971a and b; Cochran *et al.*, 1976).

Autologous and allogeneic reactions

If anti-tumour antibodies detected *in vitro* have relevance *in vivo* they should certainly react with autologous tumour cells. Most studies, whether examining the fixation of antibody to tumour cells, or the ability of antibody to kill such cells, have reported autologous reactions. The proportion of positive individuals varies widely, the incidence of positive reactors reflecting technical factors, the clinical stage of the patients studied, masking of target cell antigens by attached antibodies or materials such as sialic acid and perhaps the existence of subgroups of tumour antigens. Patients on (B-cell) immunosuppressive therapy may also have a reduction of tumour-directed antibody.

Less predictable has been the repeated observation that anti-tumour antibodies frequently cross react with allogeneic tumour cells of identical histogenesis. While reminiscent of the observation that animal tumours induced by the same oncogenic virus share antigens (Klein *et al.*, 1962) the narrow histological specificity observed in man is not seen in animal viral tumours and has been interpreted as indicating these antigens to be organ-specific rather than tumour-specific. This remains to be resolved.

Extensively studied tumours such as Burkitt's lymphoma and melanoma have multiple neoantigens, within the nucleus and nucleolus, in the cytoplasm and on the membrane which induce characteristic patterns of antibodies detectable at different stages of disease. In melanoma there is agreement that antibodies to cytoplasmic antigens show virtually complete cross-reactivity. There is less agreement on the reaction pattern of antibodies to membrane located antigens. Most authors have found these, too, cross reactive, but Lewis *et al.* (1969) have maintained, on the basis of a long experience of membrane immunofluorescence and absorption and serum fractionation experiments that membrane-reactive antibodies are individual-specific. Recent studies suggest that where multiple membrane reactive antibodies exist, some are cross-reactive, while others are unique to the individual.

Variations of antibodies with clinical stage

The majority of studies have found anti-tumour antibodies most frequent, or at maximum titre in early malignancy, when tumour volume is small, advancing disease being associated with a declining incidence and titre of such antibodies. The situation is complicated by observations that antibodies of different specificities are characteristic of different stages of disease and while one group may be in decline, another may be augmented.

Various explanations have been advanced to explain the stage related decline of anti-tumour antibody. The simplest is that as tumour volume increases, antibody becomes attached to tumour cells until none remains in the plasma. This "sponge" theory remains to be proved, antibody titres do rise in some patients after excision of tumour but studies of the amount of antibody Ig detachable from tumours do not support it. The presence of large amounts of tumour associated antigen circulating free or complexed to antibody in advanced malignancy may cause immunological paralysis or high zone tolerance; however the transient reappearance of tumour directed antibody after the injection of autologous irradiated cells into patients with advanced melanoma (Ikonopisov *et al.*, 1970) is against this. A curious observation is that antibody produced after the injection of tumour cells alone is transient while a more stable response follows combinations of tumour cells and BCG.

Lewis *et al.* (1971, 1973) suggest an alternative explanation for the apparent loss of antibody. They have presented evidence of the development of anti-idiotypic antibodies, similar to those in chronic inflammatory disease such as rheumatoid arthritis, in patients with advanced cancer. These are said to react with anti-tumour antibodies (and thus are anti-antibodies) rendering them undetectable. It is also possible that tumour cells alter antigenically during the progression of malignant disease as a result of selection pressures. This might be due to antigenic modulation or the emergence of clones with less emphatic antigenic structure. Selection pressures may also favour the survival of cells with marked masking of surface antigens. Cells modified in these ways would constitute a weaker immunogenic stimulus and in the absence of an appropriate continuing stimulus the immune response might decline. Evidence which may be interpreted as supporting this comes from the observation that tumour-directed antibodies are less detectable in patients who remain tumour-free for substantial periods.

Tumour directed antibodies in cancer contacts

Anti-tumour antibodies are increased in the families of patients with neuroblastoma (Hellström *et al.*, 1968) and in the relatives and close associates of sarcoma patients (Morton and Malmgren, 1968; Eilber and Morton, 1970). Further studies of cell-mediated and humoral immunity have shown tumour-sensitisation in environmental contacts of patients with osteogenic sarcoma (Priori *et al.*, 1971; Byers *et al.*, 1975; Boddie *et al.*, 1975; Singh *et al.*, 1977), neuroblastoma (Graham-Pole *et al.*, 1976), the leukaemias (Levine *et al.*, 1972; Hilberg *et al.*, 1973), Burkitt lymphoma (Cochran *et al.*, 1973) and breast carcinoma (Byers *et al.*, 1975). Contact reactions are apparently identical with those in tumour patients and have been interpreted as indicating a horizontally transmitted immunogenic agent. This is reminiscent of the situation revealed by studies of cat leukaemia virus (FeLV) (Hardy *et al.*, 1976). Virus exposed cats show a variety of results, in part related to the dose of FeLV encountered, but also reflecting host resistance, which in turn depends upon genetic factors, metabolic factors such as nutritional status, age at exposure and the extent, duration, degree and timing of any previous exposure to FeLV. A minority of cats develop leukaemia, others, auto-immune diseases such as autoimmune haemolytic anaemia, while the majority develop antibodies to FeLV and a relative resistance to this virus. While knowledge of comparable human carcinogens is rudimentary, studies of clusters of malignancy (Vianna *et al.*, 1971) or sensitisation seem potentially instructive.

Antibody dependent cell-mediated cytotoxicity

Antibody molecules attached to tumour cells, even at low concentration, make these cells susceptible to killing by mononuclear cells which are not specifically reactive (in an immunological sense) with tumour associated antigens (Möller, 1965; McLennan and Loewi, 1968). A variety of cells including granulocytes, macrophages and B lymphocytes can kill antibody primed target cells, but interest has focused recently on an apparently separate population of intermediate sized lymphocytes (K cells) which are specially active in this situation. K cells are not fully characterised but can be identified by several characteristics including, non-adherence to glass or plastic, lack of phagocytic activity, receptors for the Fc portion of IgG, inability to form rosettes with sheep erythrocytes, independence of thymic influence and sensitivity to azathioprine (McLennan, 1976). K cells have been shown to kill antibody-primed animal tumour cells (Skurzak *et al.*, 1972; Pollack *et al.*, 1972) and human cancer cells, including leukaemia cells (Hersey *et al.*, 1973) bladder cancer cells (O'Toole *et al.*, 1973) and melanoma cells (Kodera and Bean, 1975). Their cytotoxic activity appears to depend on their capacity to attach by a specific receptor to the Fc portion of antibody molecules.

Much remains to be learned about this system, but its actual importance in the natural control of tumours and potential utility in passive immunotherapy seems likely to be considerable.

TUMOUR CELL ASSOCIATED IMMUNOGLOBULINS

Antibody to tumour associated antigens might reasonably be expected to attach to tumour cells *in vivo* and be detectable on such cells. Support for the possibility of adsorption of antibodies to tumour cells *in vivo* comes from reports of detection of circulating anti-tumour antibody only *after tumour removal* (Pilch and Riggins, 1966; Gold, 1967). Several authors have found immunoglobulins in tumour extracts (Anthony and Parsons, 1965; Witz and Ran, 1970; Cox and Romsdahl, 1973), mainly IgG but with some IgA. Others have separated Ig from tumour cells by low pH elution (Witz and Ran, 1970; Thunold *et al.*, 1973; Vanky *et al.*, 1976), a standard technique for dissociating antibody from antigen. Tumour tissue comprises a variety of cells, including Ig secreting lymphoid cells (Kopf *et al.*, 1966) and Ig in extracts of cytologically unfractionated tumour tissue cannot be regarded as

3. Immunological Responses Against Tumour Cells

deriving exclusively from tumour cells. Localisation of Ig in tumours has been attempted using techniques such as direct immunofluorescence with monospecific antisera against Ig subclasses with varied results. Some authors have found no tumour cell associated Ig (Kopf et al., 1966; Nairn et al., 1971a and b) and others a relatively high incidence of tumour cells coated with Ig (Gutterman et al., 1973; Izsak et al., 1974; Vanky et al., 1976), especially in tumours of relatively high malignancy. It is probable, though unproved, that some of this Ig is anti-tumour antibody although non-specific attachment of globulins to cells can occur (Ishizaka, 1963). Proof that eluted Ig are tumour-directed antibodies would require that they specifically (re)attach to the appropriate tumour cells; a technically difficult task.

It is also necessary to explain why only a proportion of tumour cells have Ig attached. Various explanations for this have been advanced.

(a) In advanced disease a decline in antibody production may provide insufficient antibody molecules to coat each tumour cell.

(b) Low avidity antibody may be removed by even gentle preparative techniques.

(c) Antibody penetration into solid tumours is poor. Experiments with isotope-labelled antibody show circulating tumour cells and cells in ascitic fluid to be better labelled than those in solid tumours (Witz et al., 1969; Witz and Ran, 1970).

(d) Lysosomal proteolytic enzymes, known to exist free around cells, may cleave cell-associated Ig molecules leaving only part attached to the cell membrane (Keisari and Witz, 1975). Indicator antisera directed mainly against the cleaved portion would not then detect the attached fragments. The need for caution in selection of indicator antisera, and in interpretation of both positive and negative findings is apparent.

Even greater caution is necessary in assessing the significance of Ig associated with lymphomas and leukaemias. B lymphocytes (thymus independent or bursa-equivalent derived) produce surface Ig molecules which are integrated into the plasma membrane, such structures being absent from T lymphocytes (thymus-derived). Such markers, and others (Chapter 6) have been used to classify normal lymphocytes and the cells of lymphoid malignancies (Greaves et al., 1976; Brouet et al., 1976; Belpomme et al., 1976). Before an assignment is made, it must be established by techniques such as serial elution (Foulis et al., 1973) that the Ig is structural and not specifically or non-specifically attached Ig.

The simple studies have been to some extent completed and antibodies with at least relative tumour specificity identified in patients with many different cancers. The more difficult task of ascertaining the true specificity of the antibodies remains largely untouched. Few studies bear comparison with the extensive and meticulously careful analysis of anti-tumour antibodies in Burkitt's lymphoma patients and most lack adequate analysis of organ or foetal specificity, of variations of antibody titre with crucial clinical events, and of cross blocking by allogeneic sera from patients with similar or dissimilar tumours. The past decade has yielded a broad and superficial advance in our knowledge of humoral immunity to tumour cells, which is a necessary prelude to the difficult in-depth studies in prospect. The advent and extension of newer and less subjective techniques such as the radio-immunoassay and the enzyme-linked immune adsorbent assay is thus timely and seems likely to expedite the necessary studies.

The role of anti-tumour antibody *in vivo* remains unclear. Some of the phenomena detected *in vitro*, agglutination, opsonisation, immune adherence, inhibition of tumour cell motility, complement dependent cytotoxicity and antibody dependent cell-mediated cytotoxicity, *if active in vivo and not merely laboratory artefacts*, could have an adverse effect on tumour cell survival, multiplication and spread. Others, such as blocking of effector cells and enhancement of tumour growth (Chapter 5) would appear unfavourable to the host. As all these activities may well be concurrent the task of assessing the role and significance of anti-tumour antibodies is daunting and perhaps impossible. For some years anti-tumour antibodies were cast as the villains of the tumour immunology scene. This, like most generalisations, is certainly an oversimplification and the important requirement, from a clinical standpoint, is to identify those specific situations in which antibody-mediated effects may be deleterious.

Cell Mediated Immunity to Tumour Associated Antigens

Tumour associated antigens, unique to tumour cells or present on tumour cells but absent from normal *adult* cells may cause tumour tissue to be handled as a (weak) allograft. If this is the case, by analogy with true allografts and xenografts, cell-mediated immune mechanisms are likely to be more important than humoral immunity in the induction of rejection. With this in mind many studies *in vivo* and *in vitro* have been concerned with cell-mediated tumour-directed immunity (CMI).

STUDIES *IN VIVO*

Skin reactivity to tumour materials
It is established practice to test for delayed hypersensitivity in certain infectious diseases by the intradermal injection of antigenic material from the appropriate organism, the tuberculin and lepromin tests being well known examples of this. On theoretical grounds this type of technique has much to commend it in comparison with *in vitro* assays. A positive reaction

requires that the various components of the cellular immune response be intact and that they function sequentially and in correct order. Such tests assess the phagocytic and antigen processing capacity of macrophages, the memory function of specifically sensitised lymphocytes, the capacity of antigenically stimulated lymphocytes to release lymphokines and the ability of such lymphokines to attract, retain and modify sufficient macrophages and lymphocytes. By comparison *in vitro* tests generally examine only one component in this series of events, which limits their value and makes interpretation difficult. However, the compendiousness of the systems examined in a skin test means that failure of one component leads to a negative result. The task is then to assess whether negativity represents non-sensitisation or merely some functional inadequacy of the mechanics of the immune response. Paradoxically, ultimate interpretation of a negative skin test would best be undertaken using concurrent *in vitro* tests to assess the integrity of each step of the reaction.

Studies *in vivo* attempting to demonstrate tuberculin-type delayed hypersensitivity skin reactions to tumour cells and tumour cell fractions have demonstrated that a proportion of cancer patients react to both autologous and allogeneic tumour material but emphasise the considerable complexity of the system. An early study by Hughes and Lytton (1964) found skin reactions to tumour materials more frequent in cancer patients than in controls, an observation confirmed by Stewart (1969a) who in a study of breast cancer found reactivity most frequent in women whose cancers were heavily infiltrated by lymphocytes (Stewart, 1969b). Subsequent studies using a variety of tumour preparations have found similar selective reactivity in a range of cancers (Table 3.3).

Table 3.3.

Some reports of skin test reactivity to tumour materials

Tumour	Reference
Acute leukaemia/BL[a]	Herberman *et al.* (1974) *Cancer Res.* **34**, 1222
Breast cancer	Stewart (1969) *Cancer (Philad.)* **23**, 1368
Breast cancer	Hollinshead *et al.* (1974) *Cancer Res.* **34**, 2961
Burkitt's lymphoma	Bluming *et al.* (1971) *Clin. exp. Immunol.* **9**, 713
Carcinoma cervix	Wells *et al.* (1973) *Surg. Gynec. Obstet.* **136**, 717
Leukaemia/carcinoma	Oren and Herberman (1971) *Clin. exp. Immunol.* **9**, 45
Lung cancer	Adkins (1973) *J. Thorac. Cardiovasc. Surg.* **66**, 557
Lung cancer/CC[a]	Wells *et al.* (1973) *Nat. Cancer Inst. Monogr.* **37**, 197
Lung cancer	Hollinshead *et al.* (1974) *J. nat. Cancer Inst.* **52**, 327
Melanoma	Fass *et al.* (1970) *Lancet* **1**, 116
Melanoma	Mavligit *et al.* (1973) *Nat. Cancer Inst. Monogr.* **37**, 167
NPC[a]	Levine *et al.* (1976) *Int. J. Cancer* **17**, 155
Various cancers	Hughes and Lytton (1964) *Brit. med. J.* **1**, 209

[a]NPC = nasopharyngeal carcinoma, BL = Burkitt's lymphoma, CC = carcinoma of cervix.

The need for caution in interpretation and for simultaneous tests with control materials is highlighted by the experience of Fass and his colleagues (Fass *et al.*, 1970). These workers skin tested African melanoma patients with melanoma materials and found a high incidence of apparently very specific reactions, however an extension of the study, using control preparations of skin, showed the reactivity to be much less melanoma-specific.

We have skin tested melanoma patients with autologous irradiated (or formalinised) tumour cells prior to the use of the preparations in active specific immunotherapy and found about half the patients positive. An example of the type of reaction obtained is shown in Figure 3.1. Positivity or negativity did not, however, correlate with prognosis.

Recent studies have reported the use of preparations of melanoma antigens, rendered relatively pure by enzymatic digestion, salt extraction, column separation and electrophoresis (Hollinshead *et al.*, 1974; Sega *et al.*, 1976). Professor Hollinshead has extracted several apparently unique tumour associated antigens from each tumour which has been examined. These antigens vary in their capacity to evoke positive skin tests, some being considerably more active and specific than the relatively crude membrane preparations previously available. This is partly explained by inhibitors of skin reactivity which are also extractable from tumour cell membranes and in cruder preparations may prevent a reaction to the potentially active tumour antigens present.

The potential for purified antigens in cancer diagnosis and serial monitoring of cancer patients would seem considerable and their utility in these roles is currently under intensive investigation.

Skin window technique

In this approach (Rebuck and Crowley, 1955) the skin is abraded by fine sandpaper and a glass coverslip applied. Cells move from the underlying tissues onto the coverslip and may be identified and counted after fixation and staining (Fig. 3.2). Serial samples on separate coverslips are usually taken between 6 and 48 hours and the composition of the cell population is observed to change during this time. The initial population consists almost exclusively of polymorphonuclear leucocytes, later it changes to include macrophages, lymphòcytes, basophils and occasional eosinophils. Dizon and Southam (1963) found reduced macrophage emigration in patients with advanced cancer; the reduction correlating well with the patient's physical condition but not with radiotherapy or chemotherapy. Most patients with localised cancer had macrophage emigration similar to normal individuals.

Black and Leis (1970, 1971, 1973) modified the technique for the study of tumour directed cellular hypersensitivity in breast cancer by placing cryostat

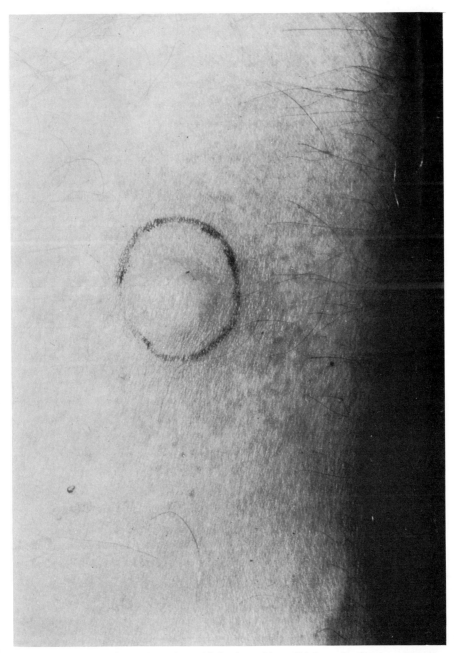

Fig. 3.1. Skin reaction to intradermal injection of 1×10^6 formalin fixed autologous melanoma cells in a patient with melanoma spread to the regional lymph nodes.

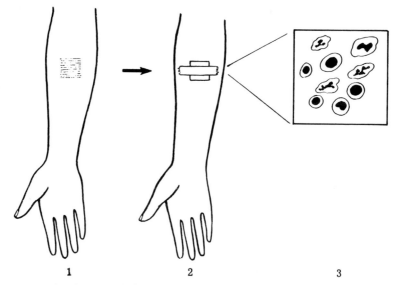

Fig. 3.2. Skin window technique.

1. Volar epidermis abraded by fine grade sandpaper.
2. Coverslip (with or without cryostat section) applied to abraded area by adhesive tape.
3. Coverslip removed, stained and attached cells identified and counted.

sections of breast cancer or benign breast conditions on the coverslip in contact with the abrasion. They report special macrophage and basophil reactions to autologous cancer sections, in around 40% of cancer patients and similar reactions to autologous tissue in under 10% of patients with non-malignant breast disease. A positive reaction in the cancer patients correlated with localised disease, peritumoral lymphocytic infiltration and axillary node sinus histiocytosis, features previously shown to be associated with a favourable prognosis (page 23).

This interesting technique has been surprisingly little exploited, perhaps reflecting a lack of enthusiasm for the cytological interpretation of mixed cell populations.

TESTS TO ASSESS TUMOUR-DIRECTED CELL MEDIATED IMMUNITY *IN VITRO*

Most studies of tumour-directed cellular immunity have used *in vitro* techniques which purport to measure aspects of the cellular response and reflect delayed hypersensitivity *in vivo*. These fall into three broad categories:

(*1*) tests measuring the effects of materials (lymphokines) released from antigen-stimulated sensitised lymphocytes

(2) tests in which putatively sensitised lymphocytes are exposed to tumour cells or tumour cell extracts and assessed for evidence of specific blast transformation

(3) tests in which a specific effector function is sought by looking for lymphocyte-mediated inhibition of target cell growth or target cell destruction. Where experimental design involves antigenic recognition the activity of both afferent and efferent limbs of the immune response may be assayed simultaneously.

Antigen triggered production of lymphokines

The leucocyte migration inhibition technique (LMT). This was devised by Søborg and Bendixen in 1967 from the macrophage migration technique of George and Vaughan (1962). Blood leucocytes are mixed with tumour cells or tumour cell extracts, and the production of inhibitory activity assessed either as a one stage capillary assay (Fig. 3.3), the leucocyte population

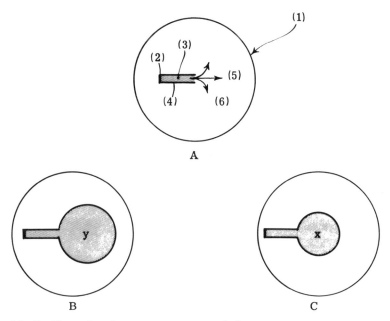

Fig. 3.3. *Capillary migration assay*, one stage technique.

A. Schema of migration assay. (1) Tissue culture vessel. (2) Clay seal at end of capillary. (3) Peripheral blood leucocytes ± tumour antigen. (4) Capillary tube. (5) Direction of migration of leucocytes. (6) Tissue culture medium + 10% foetal calf serum.

B. Representative migration area in medium without added tumour antigen.

C. Inhibited leucocyte migration area in presence of tumour antigens. Inhibition is quantified by dividing x by y.

acting as both the source of the inhibitory materials and the indicator system, or as a two-step assay (Spitler, 1973), the supernatants of lymphocyte/ tumour cultures being assayed for inhibitory activity on allogeneic normal leucocytes or xenogeneic macrophages (Fig. 3.4). The two step assay permits the simultaneous assessment of the production of lymphokines other than migration inhibition factor (MIF) in appropriate indicator systems. It may also be used to examine populations of cells which are less actively motile than peripheral leucocytes (e.g. peritumoral lymphoid cells).

The LMT was first applied to human malignant disease by Andersen *et al.* (1970) in a study of women with breast cancer. Numerous reports have since been published establishing the usefulness and limitations of this technique (Table 3.4). The technique is relatively simple and in our experience readily mastered and the necessary equipment uncomplicated and inexpensive. The one-stage capillary assay is rather cumbersome and attempts have been made to simplify the technique, the best to date being that of Clausen (1971) who places leucocytes and antigen in wells in an agarose plate and measures the radial movement of the leucocytes in the space between the agarose and the

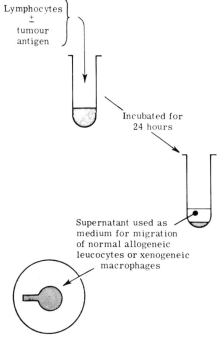

Fig. 3.4. Two stage leucocyte migration assay. Inhibition is assessed by comparing normal leucocyte or macrophage migration in supernatant of lymphocytes plus tumour antigen with that in supernatant of lymphocytes alone.

Table 3.4.

Some reports of leucocyte migration techniques in the assessment of tumour-directed cell mediated immunity

Tumour	Reference
Breast cancer	Andersen et al. (1970) Int. J. Cancer **5**, 357
Breast cancer	Cochran et al. (1973) Brit. J. Cancer **28**, Suppl. 1, 77
Breast cancer	McCoy et al. (1974) J. nat. Cancer Inst. **53**, 11
Breast cancer ⎫ Colon cancer ⎭	Tautz and Ax (1974) Z. Immun-Forsch **147**, 155
Carcinoma cervix	Goldstein et al. (1971) Amer. J. Obstet. Gynec. **111**, 751
Carcinoma cervix	Chen (1975) Amer. J. Obstet. Gynec. **121**, 91
Colorectal cancer	Guillou and Giles (1973) Gut **14**, 733
Colorectal cancer	Elias and Elias (1975) Surg. Forum **24**, 131
Lung cancer	Boddie et al. (1975) Int. J. Cancer **15**, 823
Lymphomas	Braun et al. (1972) Blood **39**, 368
Malignant melanoma	Cochran et al. (1972) Brit. med. J. **4**, 67
Malignant melanoma	McCoy et al. (1975) J. nat. Cancer Inst. **55**, 19
Neuroblastoma	Graham-Pole et al. (1976) Lancet **2**, 1376
Renal carcinoma	Kjaer, M. (1975) Europ. J. Cancer **11**, 281
Various	Segall et al. (1972) Int. J. Cancer **9**, 417

plate base (Fig. 3.5). This technique in which tuberculin was initially used as antigen, has now been successful in studies of human cancer (Spitler, 1973; Ax and Tautz, 1974). Another useful variant is the agatose droplet technique (Harrington and Stastny, 1973).

There is little unanimity as to what constitutes the best antigenic preparation for use in LMTs. Information on the exact nature of the antigens being detected and on the role, if any, of foetal antigens are particularly pressing needs. There is evidence that the effect is due to release of a soluble mediator from lymphocytes but whether it acts exclusively against macrophages (monocytes) or also against granulocytes, or whether separate lymphokines act on different cell populations is not known (Ross et al., 1978).

Leucocyte adherence inhibition (LAI) assay. In 1972 Halliday and Miller reported that glass adherent mouse leucocytes lost adherence in an immunologically specific manner in the presence of tumour extracts (Fig. 3.6). The technique was performed on haemocytometer plates and involved tricky manoeuvres to remove the coverslip and wash the cell bearing surface. Despite this Halliday and associates used it successfully in the immuno-diagnosis of hepatocellular carcinoma (Halliday et al., 1974), and in studies of colorectal and breast carcinoma (Maluish and Halliday, 1974) and melanoma (Halliday et al., 1975). These observations have been confirmed,

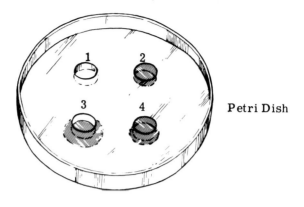

Petri Dish

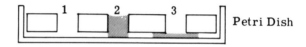

Petri Dish

Fig. 3.5. Clausen migration technique.
Leucocytes with or without tumour antigen (2) are placed in holes cut in an agarose plate (1). After 24 hours incubation the area of migration of the leucocytes in the space between the agarose and the base of the plate is measured. Migration is compared in the presence (4) and absence (3) of tumour antigen.

but the tendency has been to simplify the technique by electronic rather than visual cell counting (Lampert and Deitmair, 1973), by performing the test in glass tubes rather than on haemocytometer slides (Hólan *et al.*, 1974; Grosser and Thomson, 1975) and by using purified mononuclear cells (Powell *et al.*, 1975).

It was initially held that the mechanism of LAI was similar to that of the leucocyte migration technique, antigen stimulated sensitised lymphocytes releasing a factor which reduced leucocyte adherence to glass. However, Marti *et al.* (1976) using a tube LAI technique presented evidence that decreased adherence may be due to interactions of cytophilic IgG antibody with leucocytes.

Mazuran *et al.* (1976) have described a technique in which monocyte spreading on glass is inhibited by tumour extracts. The technique, which sounds relatively uncomplicated, has similarities to the LAI technique. Confirmation of the accuracy and value of this test are awaited.

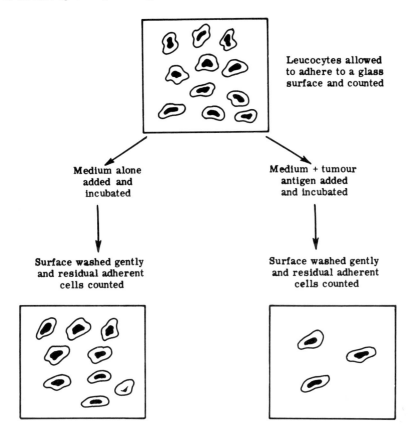

Fig. 3.6. Leucocyte adherence inhibition assay. The proportion of leucocytes adherent after exposure to tumour antigen is related to that adherent after exposure to medium alone or control antigens.

Macrophage electrophoretic mobility test. Field and Caspary (1970) described this technique in which lymphocytes, guinea pig peritoneal macrophages and tissue extracts (white matter of brain, cancerous tissue or other organs) are incubated together and the passive migration of individual macrophages in the electric field of a cytopherometer is measured. The technique was initially exploited by Field and his collaborators (Caspary, 1972; Field *et al.*, 1973) who claimed a high degree of discrimination of cancer patients with it. Confirmatory results have now come from several groups including Pritchard *et al.* (1972) and Light *et al.* (1975). However, there are also contrary studies in which discrimination between cancer patients and controls was not demonstrated (Lewkonia *et al.*, 1974; Crozier *et al.*, 1976). Most workers have found the technique difficult and capricious and record major operational problems. A common difficulty is the provision of suitable

xenogeneic macrophages (Field and Shenton, 1975), which may apparently
be overcome by the use of human granulocytes (Preece and Light, 1976) or
tanned sheep erythrocytes (Porzsolt et al., 1975). A more detailed review of
the macrophage electrophoretic mobility test and its modifications may be
found in a recent leading article in the Lancet (1976).

Lymphocyte blastogenesis by tumour materials

Theoretical considerations require a sensitised lymphocyte confronted with
the sensitising antigen to undergo blast transformation prior to mitosis and
clonal expansion. It is therefore logical to expose cancer patients'
lymphocytes to tumour antigens and look for transformation. This technique
has been successfully applied (Table 3.5) but many workers find it difficult,
due to the considerable variability of transformation systems, and the low
level of transformation induced by tumour antigen, possibly reflecting the
small proportion of lymphocytes likely to be responsive to any single antigen.
Using membrane preparations or formalin fixed tumour cells, we found it
unusual for stimulated lymphocytes to incorporate more than two to three
times the isotopic uptake of unstimulated cells. If these problems can be
overcome, the system is undoubtedly flexible, permitting the use of fresh
tumour cells, frozen-stored tumour cells and tumour cell extracts as
stimulating "antigens" and permitting the investigation of sera for transformation inhibiting activity (Vanky et al., 1971).

Table 3.5.

Some reports of tumour cell induced lymphocyte blastogenesis in the assessment of
tumour-directed cell mediated immunity

Tumour	Reference
Brain tumours	Brooks et al. (1972). *J. exp. Med.* **136**, 1631
Burkitt lymphoma	Golub et al. (1972). *Int. J. Cancer* **10**, 157
Carcinoma	Stjernswärd et al. (1968). *E. Afr. Med. J.* **45**, 484
Carcinoma	Watkins et al. (1971). *Nature (New Biol.)* **231**, 83
Colon cancer ⎫ Leukaemia ⎭	Mavligit et al. (1973). *Nature (New Biol.)* **243**, 188
Kaposi's sarcoma	Taylor et al. (1971). *Int. J. Cancer* **8**, 468
Leukaemia	Bach et al. (1969). *Science* **166**, 1520
Leukaemia	Fridman and Kourilsky (1969). *Nature* **224**, 277
Leukaemia	Gutterman et al. (1972). *Cancer Res.* **342**, 2524
Melanoma	Jehn et al. (1970). *New Engl. J. Med.* **283**, 329
Melanoma	Nagel et al. (1970). *Cancer Res.* **30**, 1828
Sarcomas ⎫ Carcinomas ⎭	Vanky et al. (1971). *Israel J. med. Sci.* **7**, 211
Sarcomas ⎫ Carcinomas ⎪ Brain tumours ⎪ Myeloma ⎭	Vanky et al. (1976) *In* "Clinical Tumour Immunology" (Wybran and Staquet, Eds.) 55-68. Pergamon Press, Oxford

Technical aspects of the test are covered by Vanky *et al*. (1976) who stress the need for full control studies and the use of dose-response curves. The development of some means of amplifying the specific response would greatly increase the utility of this theoretically attractive but practically limited technique.

Tests measuring tumour target cell killing and growth inhibition

If tumour directed immunity is significant in the control of malignant disease the demonstration of lymphocyte sensitisation is not enough; it is necessary to show that lymphocytes, or their products or cells modified by and acting under the influence of lymphocytes or their products are capable of killing tumour cells or severely restricting their growth. This crucial requirement explains the widespread and continuing interest in techniques which demonstrate lymphocyte killing or growth inhibition of tumour target cells *in vitro*. If selective killing is demonstrable *in vitro* it is arguable, though difficult of proof, that the same cells might act similarly *in vivo*.

Because of the crucial importance of an effector activity of the immune response against tumour cells, these techniques have been very widely exploited and the success and frustrations of those active in this area are a salutary warning to researchers involved with other techniques. It is possible, though not certain, that other methods, such as LAI and LMT, will present similar problems when subjected to the meticulous scrutiny to which the cytotoxicity assays have been exposed.

Cytotoxicity has involved all levels of scientific endeavour from molecular biology, directed to elucidating the molecular alterations in the cell membrane which lead to cytolysis, to attempts to apply the techniques to the routine assessment of cancer patients. Many studies have been well conceived and executed, the problems encountered reflecting limitations of the available technology. However, the claims from a minority of studies take little account of lymphocyte heterogeneity and of the vagaries of tissue cultured cells.

The initial technique was the colony inhibition technique devised by Ingegerd Hellström in a mouse sarcoma system (Hellström and Sjögren, 1965). Cultured colonies of replicating tumour cells and of non-tumour cells were exposed to lymphocytes from tumorous and control animals and the number of colonies surviving lymphocyte confrontation were counted after three to five days. This proved a productive and very useful technique. Selective tumour cell colony inhibiting activity was demonstrated in animal systems and with lymphocytes from patients with neuroblastoma (Hellström *et al*., 1968), melanomas, sarcomas and cancers of colon, kidney, lung, skin and female breast (Hellström *et al*., 1968, 1970, 1971). The test is technically demanding and few laboratories have been willing or able to establish it for routine use, most preferring to investigate the relatively simpler assays available from 1970 onwards.

Takasugi and Klein (1970) cultured tumour cells or control cells in multi-chamber plates and after a period to allow attachment to the plate exposed them to tumour bearer and control lymphocytes. After coculture with the lymphocytes, detached target cells and cell debris were washed out of the chambers, the residual attached cells fixed, stained and counted manually. The number of target cells surviving exposure to tumour bearer lymphocytes was then related to the number surviving control lymphocyte contact. A similar technique which employed culture plates with larger chambers, permitting better cell dispersal and the deployment of higher ratios of lymphocytes, was introduced by Hellström et al. (1971).

Initial studies indicated that patients with a variety of malignancies had lymphocytes which were selectively cytotoxic for cultured tumour cells histogenetically similar to their own tumour (Table 3.6). A weak point of these methods, was the need for time consuming and exacting visual counting of residual target cells. Attempts have been made to avoid this by the use of image analysers (Takasugi et al., 1973a) or by isotopic labelling of the target cells before or after exposure to the effector cells (Bean et al., 1973; Oldham and Herberman, 1973). These alternative techniques provide considerable advantages and have been increasingly adopted.

Table 3.6.

Some reports of cytotoxicity techniques in the assessment of tumour-directed cell mediated immunity

Tumour	Reference
Bladder cancer	Bubenik et al. (1970). Int. J. Cancer **5**, 39
Bladder cancer	O'Toole et al. (1972). Int. J. Cancer **10**, 77
Brain tumours	Kumar et al. (1973). Brit. J. Cancer **28**, Suppl. 1, 135
Breast cancer	Fossati et al. (1972). Int. J. Cancer **10**, 391
Breast cancer	Avis et al. (1974). J. nat. Cancer Inst. **52**, 1041
Carcinoma cervix	Vasudevan et al. (1970). Int. J. Cancer **6**, 506
Colon cancer	Nairn et al. (1971). Brit. med. J. **4**, 706
Colon cancer	Baldwin et al. (1973). Int. J. Cancer **12**, 84
Lung cancer	Pierce and deVald (1975). Cancer Res. **35**, 3577
Lung cancer	Vose et al. (1975). Int. J. Cancer **15**, 308
Melanoma	Fossati et al. (1971). Int. J. Cancer **8**, 344
Melanoma	deVries et al. (1972). Int. J. Cancer **9**, 567
Neuroblastoma ⎱ Renal cancer ⎰	Kumar et al. (1972). Int. J. Cancer **10**, 36
Osteosarcomas	Cohen et al. (1973). J. nat. Cancer Inst. **50**, 585
Renal cancer	Diehl et al. (1971). Int. J. Cancer **7**, 277
Skin cancer	Nairn et al. (1971). Brit. med. J. **4**, 701

Technical problems have been overshadowed by the realisation that cytotoxicity measured in this way was not as tumour-specific as had at first been claimed. Admirably thorough investigation of all aspects of the techniques has indicated that the results obtained can vary dramatically according to the source of lymphocytes, the methods and degree of preparation and purification of the lymphocytes, characteristics of the target tumour cells such as duration in culture, growth rate, adhesiveness to plastic and labelling qualities and the method of performance of all the many steps of the technique. This topic is fully discussed in recent publications (Bloom and David, 1976; Baldwin and Embleton, 1976).

In order to be effective in tumour control *in vivo*, the immune apparatus must have some capacity to kill tumour cells or severely restrain their growth. On the basis of extensive studies of transplantation immunology and the tumour immunology of experimental animals, the lymphocyte seems likely to be at least one mediator of this activity. It remains highly desirable that techniques become available to permit examination of this function. Much effort is being devoted to attempts to modify existing techniques for assessing cell mediated cytotoxicity and to devise new techniques. These efforts at present disclose a discouragingly complex situation, but the clamant need dictates that efforts must continue despite setbacks.

RESULTS OF STUDIES ASSESSING TUMOUR-DIRECTED CELL-MEDIATED IMMUNITY

In order to avoid repetition I will discuss the results of the various assays for cellular immunity together, indicating disparities of results where appropriate. The findings are broadly similar to those in studies of tumour-directed humoral immunity.

Comparisons of cancer patients and control individuals

Lymphocytes from a majority of cancer patients have been shown to be sensitised to or cytotoxic for autologous tumour cells and allogeneic tumour cells of similar histogenesis by virtually all techniques employed. The exponents of the MEM test and its modifications go further and say that all cancer patients are sensitised to "cancer basic protein", a material present in most cancers regardless of histogenesis. However, with the histological restrictions noted above, tumour-directed cellular immunity has been demonstrated by most other techniques in from 40 to 80% of cancer patients and in 10 to 25% of clinically tumour-free control individuals. Reactions against autologous and homologous tumour cells are similarly frequent. As with the cross reactions observed in antibody studies this finding calls into question the nature and specificity of the antigens detected. The type of data obtained is exemplified by our own experience with LMT (Table 3.7).

Table 3.7.

The effect of autologous and allogeneic tumour cells and extracts on the migration of leucocytes from cancer patients and control donors

Type of cancer	Antigen	Leucocyte migration inhibited/Total tested					
		Autologous tests		Allogeneic tests		Control donor leucocytes	
		No.	%	No.	%	No.	%
Malignant melanoma	SN[a]	8/10	80	33/55	60	9/63	14
Malignant melanoma	FC[b]	12/15	80	87/105	83	9/61	1̀5
Breast cancer	SN[a]	18/32	56	56/106	53	24/157	15
Neuroblastoma	SN[b]	3/4	75	8/8	100	16/61	26

[a]SN is centrifuged supernatant of tumour homogenate.
[b]FC is formalin fixed single cell suspension from tumours.

The interpretation of reactions in normal individuals presents problems, which largely remain to be solved. This has been especially troublesome in studies of cell-mediated cytotoxicity. As noted above, in the earliest phase of such studies the lymphocytes of cancer patients were found to kill tumour cells preferentially. Later several workers found some control donor lymphocytes able to kill tumour cells as effectively as those of cancer patients. This was extensively investigated by Takasugi et al. (1973b) and the following facts emerged. Cultured tumour cells vary in susceptibility to killing by lymphocytes. Some selection is therefore necessary to obtain target cells suitable for the test system. Target cell susceptibility is partly a basic cellular characteristic, but may also vary with duration of culture (Takasugi et al., 1973b; deVries et al., 1974), the type of culture medium employed (Sulit et al., 1976), mycoplasma and other infections, culture density at harvest and stage of the cell cycle (Leneva and Svet-Moldavsky, 1974). These comments apply equally to non-tumour culture lines and the choice of appropriate control target cells is a distinctly emotive subject.

Lymphocytes from control donors vary in their capacity to kill cultured tumour cells. This may be T lymphocyte-mediated killing due to sensitisation of environmental contacts (Hellström et al., 1968) or laboratory workers (Takasugi, 1973b) or to transplantation antigen disparities between lymphocytes and target cells (Cerottini et al., 1970) or possibly to ethnic factors. Normal African blacks are sensitised to melanoma antigens (Tautz and Ax, 1975) and the lymphocytes of normal American blacks kill cultured melanoma cells (Hellström et al., 1973). Spontaneous cytotoxicity by normal lymphocytes has received much attention (Takasugi *et al.*, 1973b; Rosenberg, 1974). Part of this activity may be due to non-T lymphocytes and some to macrophages. Attempts have been made selectively to deplete leucocyte populations of different types of cells (see Pross and Baines, 1976 for review). Spontaneous cytotoxicity is less in cancer patients than control donors (Takasugi *et al.*, 1973b), may mask specific T cell cytotoxicity and is due in part to non-T lymphocytes with receptors for the Fc portion of Ig and complement (deVries *et al.*, 1974; Peter *et al.*, 1975). Since both tumour patients' and control donors' lymphocytes vary in terms of spontaneous and "specific" cytotoxic activity it is possible to envisage situations in which low-cytotoxic tumour-bearer lymphocytes (low to moderate specific, and low spontaneous cytotoxicity) tested against the same target cells simultaneously with highly cytotoxic control lymphocytes (nil specific, high spontaneous cytotoxicity) would kill a relatively lower proportion of tumour cells. Results obtained in this manner with heterogeneous lymphocyte populations are thus virtually uninterpretable.

Clinical stage and tumour-directed cellular immunity

A majority of reports record a stage-related decline in tumour directed cell-mediated immunity correlated with the extent of dissemination but also to some extent with tumour volume. This may be seen as a reduction in the proportion of reactive individuals or merely as a reduction in reaction strength. Table 3.8 summarises our own results in melanoma and breast carcinoma patients. While the stage relationship is clear, the major difference is between patients with limited disease (I + II) and those with disseminated disease (III). Whether this decline precedes tumour expansion or is merely a sequel to it is discussed in the section on "immunological monitoring" (*q. v.*).

The mechanisms of stage-related reduction in detectable sensitisation are incompletely understood. That it is not absolute or irreversible is shown by the (re)development of cytotoxic lymphocytes after immunisation with autologous irradiated tumour cells in patients with advanced malignancy (Currie *et al.*, 1971). Also when patients with advanced melanoma receive systemic or intralesional BCG (with or without autologous irradiated or formalinised tumour cells) the frequency of detectable LMT reactions approximates to that of patients with localised disease (Table 3.8). If immune paralysis exists in the patient with advanced malignancy, it is only partial and is remediable. High-zone tolerance cannot be excluded as causing the decline in reactivity as the tumour cells, administered in the "unnatural" form of a suspension could break tolerance. The administration of tumour cells with or without an adjuvant may also stimulate concomitant immunity (Gershon, 1974).

Another possibility is that large volumes of tumour may sequester active committed lymphocytes, removing them from the peripheral blood. Against

Table 3.8.

The frequency of leucocyte migration inhibition related to clinical stage

Cancer type and stage	Leucocyte migration inhibited/Total tested			
	SN antigens[a]		FC antigens[b]	
	No.	%	No.	%
Malignant melanoma				
Stage I	24/37	65	16/19	84
Stage II	7/15	47	21/21	100
Stage III	0/6	0	12/24	50
Stage III, immunotherapy			35/37	95
Tumour free for under 2 years	13/16	81	23/25	92
Tumour free for over 2 years	3/12	25	22/38	58
Breast carcinoma				
Stage I	32/57	56		
Stage II	20/31	65		
Stage III	6/22	27		
Local recurrence	6/10	60		

[a]SN antigens are centrifuged supernatants of homogenised tumours.
[b]FC antigens are formalinised single cell suspensions of tumours
Stage I = primary tumour only. Stage II = primary tumour + ipsilateral draining lymph nodes involved. Stage III = spread to internal viscera or remote lymph nodes.

this is the observation that lymphocytic infiltration is a hallmark of early rather than advanced tumours, although a limited number of lymphocytes might appear sparse if spread through extensive tumour. Changes may occur in tumour cells which render them less immunogenic. In the absence of continued stimulation the immune response may wane, with the production of fewer detectable sensitised cells and lesser quantities of antitumour antibodies. The memory cell population would remain and this is supported by the prompt response to immunisation with tumour cells. Reduced immunogenicity could result from antigenic alteration by modulation or selection or from masking of antigens by immunologically inert materials such as sialic acid.

The stage-related decline of antitumour immunity is probably the end result of complex interactions of some or all of the above factors, acting simultaneously or sequentially. Recent studies have highlighted the role of free tumour antigen and antigen-antibody complexes. This is discussed in Chapter 5.

Reactions in patients remaining tumour free after treatment
Tumour directed cellular immunity persists in patients remaining tumour

free during the first two years after surgical excision. Beyond this, the reaction frequency declines as the period of tumour freedom increases (Table 3.8). This is similar to observations by O'Toole *et al.* (1972) from a study of cellular immunity to bladder cancer by cytotoxicity. The decline in reactivity seems most likely to reflect a reduced *level* of immune response in the absence of continued antigenic stimulation. Serial studies are necessary to define the kinetics of this situation and relate them more precisely to clinical events, and the topic is further discussed in the section on monitoring.

Effects of treatment on cell mediated immune reactions to tumours
Surgery, chemotherapy, radiotherapy and many drugs alter lymphocyte function significantly in *in vitro* assays and seem likely to have a similar action on function *in vivo*. The administration of immunological adjuvants, tumour cell preparations and allogeneic or xenogeneic antibodies, lymphoid cells or components of such cells in attempts at "immunotherapy" also produces wide-ranging effects on lymphocytes. These effects are the subject of Chapters 7 and 8.

Cellular sensitisation of contacts of cancer patients
Specifically sensitised lymphocytes and lymphocytes cytotoxic for appropriate tumour cells are relatively frequent in environmental and professional contacts of cancer patients. The significance and implications of this have already been discussed (p. 37).

Correlation of tumour-directed immunity and histology
The most striking observation is the cross-reactivity of lymphocytes of cancer patients with histogenetically similar allogeneic tumours, indicating that some tumour antigens have determinants which are structurally similar. Certain histological and cytological characteristics may be associated with a relatively favourable prognosis. This approach has been well developed in the case of melanoma (McGovern *et al.*, 1973). Favourable outcome could be due to tumour cells characteristics, but might also result in part from a host reaction, which seems likely to have an immunological component. We studied this by relating the occurrence of tumour-directed cell mediated immunity in patients with localised melanoma to prognostically relevant histological features of their primary tumours (Mackie *et al.*, 1973) including cross-sectional profile, ulceration, histogenetic pattern, vascular invasion, mitotic activity, peritumoral lymphoid cell aggregation, cytology, and extent and distribution of melanin. Cell-mediated reactivity correlated significantly only with mitotic rate and the presence of tumour cells in vascular channels (Table 3.9). The first finding may indicate that tumour associated antigens are relatively more expressed on actively growing tumours and the second

Table 3.9.

Correlations of leucocyte migration inhibition by melanoma extracts and histological features of primary tumour

	Leucocyte Migration Test			
	No. tested	No. positive	% Positive	P value[b]
Mitotic rate				
1/5 HPF[a]	22	11	50 ⎫	
1/5 HPF-1/HPF	24	17	70 ⎬	<0.05
1/HPF or greater	21	17	81 ⎭	
Vascular invasion				
present	17	16	94 ⎫	
absent	50	30	60 ⎭	<0.01

[a]HPF = high power field ($\times$ 300).
[b]P value from Chi-squared analysis.

that critical amounts of tumour cells or their antigens must have access to lymph nodes to permit the development of a detectable response. Nairn (1971a) found a correlation between antitumour immunity and peritumoral reaction, but we were unable to demonstrate this.

This potentially productive approach has been surprisingly little exploited.

Reactivity of lymphoid cells from sources other than peripheral blood

For reasons of accessibility of test materials most studies have examined peripheral blood lymphocytes. Although the immune reaction against a tumour is undoubtedly systemic studies of other lymphoid populations would be of great interest and are essential to a balanced view. Such studies would ideally assess several different populations simultaneously. The following summarises the information available on this topic but is clearly preliminary.

Reactivity of lymph node lymphocytes. There is concern among surgeons that the excision of tumour free lymph nodes, for instance, axillary nodes at mastectomy, may be harmful (Crile, 1967). Animal studies, which might yield practical guidance in a situation where models close to the human condition are attainable, have yielded conflicting results (see Fisher, 1971 for review). Some have shown tumour progression and spread to be accelerated after lymph node excision (Alexander and Hall, 1970; Fisher and Fisher, 1972) while others have shown node excision to have little effect on tumour behaviour (Hammond and Rolley, 1970).

It was indicated in Chapter 2 that histological changes had been recorded in tumour-draining lymph nodes which were associated with a better than average prognosis (e.g. Black and Speer, 1958). The changes are those associated with reaction to antigenic challenge and in the absence of any other antigenic stimulus may be a response to tumour.

Attempts to examine the immunology of lymph node cells *in vitro* have produced conflicting results. Cells from this source have been reported as *not* showing tumour-directed immune reactivity (Nairn *et al.*, 1971a; Humphrey *et al.*, 1971; Stjernswärd *et al.*, 1972; Vanky *et al.*, 1974), while others find them tumour reactive (Geswant *et al.*, 1971; Deodhar *et al.*, 1972; Ambus *et al.*, 1974; Ellis *et al.*, 1975). Ellis *et al.* actually found axillary node cells in breast cancer more reactive than blood lymphocytes. Ambus *et al.* reported a negative correlation between blood and lymph node reactivity, which points up to the true nature of the problem. The lymphocyte population being extensively mobile, the population of cells in a lymphoid site will vary continuously as part of normal cell turnover, with stage of tumour progression and as a treatment effect. This variation must be considered in interpreting data of this kind. Animal studies suggest that initial recognition and reaction occur in the nodes nearest to the tumour and only later can sensitised cells be detected in remote nodes or spleen (Goldfarb and Hardy, 1975). Systemic immunity could be due to lymphocyte migration, spread of lymphocyte activation products or, less likely, to the dissemination of immunogenic tumour cells or shed antigens.

Reactivity of peritumoral lymphocytes. The intimate relationship between infiltrates and tumour cells shown by light microscopy and ultrastructural studies, the favourable prognosis for infiltrated tumours shown by clinico-pathological studies and maximal association of infiltrates with early tumours suggest these cells to be reactive. Unfortunately it has proved difficult to extract them in sufficient numbers and in a condition suitable for immuno-logical assessment. Studies by Nairn et al (1971a and b) of peritumoral lymphocytes in squamous carcinoma of skin, colon carcinoma and melanoma showed no specific immunological activity. More recently Hersh *et al.* (1975) reported that lymphocytes from this source responded to PHA stimulation and that although fewer cells were obtainable from secondary tumours, cells from this source reacted better to PHA than those from primary tumours. Preliminary studies, employing rosetting techniques or the demonstration of surface Ig have shown both T and B lymphocytes although the former usually predominate.

INDICES OF CONTINUING IMMUNE RESPONSES

In the presence of a continuing immune response it may be possible to detect antigen-antibody complexes and complement consumption. This approach has proved disappointing in tumour immunology. Techniques for detecting immune complexes are intricate and not really suitable for routine application. Complement abnormalities occur in cancer patients but are neither constant nor certainly attributable to tumour antigen-antibody interactions. These topics are further discussed in Chapters 5 and 6.

References

Ablin, R. J. and Soanes, W. A. (1971). *Ann. Clin. Res.* **3**, 226.
Alexander, P. and Hall, J. (1970). *Adv. Cancer Res.* **13**, 37.
Ambus, U., Mavligit, G. M., Gutterman, J. U., McBride, C. M. and Hersh, E. M. (1974). *Int. J. Cancer* **14**, 291-300.
Andersen, V., Bjerrum, O., Bendixen, G., Schiødt, T. and Dissing, I. (1970). *Int. J. Cancer* **5**, 357.
Anthony, H. and Parsons, M. (1965). *Nature* **206**, 275-276.
Arata, I., Ogawa, I. and Tanaka, Y. (1969). *Gann.* **60**, 649.
Gann. **60**, 649.
Ax, W. and Tautz, C. (1974). *Behring Inst. Mitt.* **54**, 72-80.
Baldwin, R. W. and Embleton, M. J. (1976). *Int. Rev. exptl. Path.* **17**, 49.
Bean, M. A., Pees, H., Rosen, G. and Oettgen, H. F. (1973). *Nat. Cancer Inst. Monogr.* **37**, 41.
Belpomme, D., Dantchev, D., Joseph, R., Santoro, A., Feuilhade, DeChauvin, F., Lelarge, N., Grandjon, D., Pontvert, D. and Mathé, G. (1976). *In* "Clinical Tumour Immunology" (J. Wybran and M. J. Staquet, Eds.) 131-144. Pergamon Press, Oxford.
Black, M. M. and Speer, F. D. (1958). *Surg. Gynec Obstet.* **106**, 163-175.
Black, M. M. and Leis, H. P. (1970). *N.Y. State J. Med.* **70**, 2583-2588.
Black, M. M. and Leis, H. P. (1971). *Cancer (Philad)* **28**, 268-273.
Black, M. M. and Leis, H. P. (1973). *Cancer (Philad)* **32**, 384-389.
Bloom, E. T., Fahey, J. L., Peterson, I. A., Geering, G., Bernhard, M. and Trempe, G. (1973). *Int. J. Cancer* **12**, 21-31.
Bloom, B. R. and David, J. R. (1976). "*In vitro* methods in cell-mediated and tumor immunity". Academic Press, New York and London.
Boddie, A. W., Urist, M. M., Townsend, C., Holmes, E. C. and Morton, D. L. *Surg. Forum 1975* **26**, 154.
Brouet, J. C., Preud'homme, J. L. and Seligmann, M. (1976). *In* "Clinical Tumour Immunology" J. Wybran and M. J. Staquet, Eds.) 123-130. Pergamon Press, Oxford.
Burnham, T. K. (1972). *Lancet* **2**, 436-437.
Byers, V. S., Levin, A. S., Hackett, A. J. and Fudenberg, H. H. (1975). *J. Clin. Invest.* **55**, 500.
Caspary, E. A. (1972). *Proc. roy. Soc. Med.* **65**, 636.
Cerottini, J.-C., Nordin, A. A. and Brunner, K. T. (1970). *Nature* **228**, 1308.
Clausen, J. E. (1971). *Acta Allergol.* **26**, 56.
Cochran, A. J. (1971). *Europ. J. Clin. Biol. Res.* **16**, 44-47.
Cochran, A. J., Klein, E. and Kiessling, R. (1972). *J. nat. Cancer Inst.* **48**, 1657-1661.
Cochran, A. J., Kiessling, R. Gunvén, P., Klein, E., Johansson, B. and Foulis, A. (1973). *J. nat. Cancer Inst.* **51**, 1109-1111.
Cochran, A. J., Klein, G., Kiessling, R. and Gunven, P. (1973). *J. nat. Cancer Inst.* **51**, 1431-1436.

Cochran, A. J., Mackie, R. M., Grant, R. M., Ross, C. E., Connell, M. D., Sandilands, G., Whaley, K., Hoyle, D. E. and Jackson, A. M. (1976). *Int. J. Cancer* **18**, 298-309.

Cochran, A. J. *In* Immunological Aspects of Cancer" (1978) (J. E. Castro Ed.) 219-266. Medical and Technical Published Co. London.

Cox, I. S. and Romsdahl, M. M. (1973). *Pigment Cell* **1**, 372-381.

Crile, G. (1967). *J. Amer. Med. Ass.* **199**, 736-738.

Crozier, E. H., Hollinger, M. E., Woodend, B. E. and Robertson, J. H. (1976). *J. Clin. Path.* **29**, 608.

Currie, G. A., Lejeune, F. and Fairley, G. H. (1971). *Brit. med. J.* **2**, 305-310.

Currie, G. A. and Sime, G. C. (1973). *Nature New Biol.* **241**, 284.

Deodhar, S., Crile, G. and Esseltyn, C. (1972). *Cancer (Philad)* **28**, 1321-1325.

deVries, J. E., Cornain, S. and Rümke, P. (1974). *Int. J. Cancer* **14**, 427.

deVries, J. E., Cornain, S. and Rümke, P. (1975). *Behring Inst. Mitt.* **56**, 148-156.

Dizon, Q. S. and Southam, C. M. (1963). *Cancer (Philad)* **16**, 1288-1292.

Ehrenfeld, E. H., Gery, I. and Davis, A. M. (1961). *Lancet* **1**, 1138.

Eilber, F. R. and Morton, D. L. (1970). *Cancer (Philad)* **26**, 588.

Ellis, R. J., Wernick, G., Zabriskie, J. B. and Goldman, H. (1975). *mCancer (Philad)* **35**, 655-659.

Fagraeus, A. and Epsmark, Å. (1961). *Nature* **190**, 370.

Fass, L., Herberman, R. B., Ziegler, J. L. and Kiryabwire, J. W. M. (1970). *Lancet* **1**, 116-118.

Field, E. J. and Caspary, E. A. (1970). *Lancet* **2**, 1337-1341.

Field, E. J., Caspary, E. A. and Smith, K. S. (1973). *Brit. J. Cancer* **28**, Suppl. 1, 208.

Field, E. J. and Shenton, B. K. (1975). *IRCS Med. Sci.* **3**, 583.

Fisher, B. (1971). *Adv. Surg.* **5**, 189-259.

Fisher, B. and Fisher, E. R. (1972). *Cancer (Philad)* **29**, 1496-1501.

Foulis, A. K., Cochran, A. J. and Anderson, J. R. (1973). *Clin. exp. Immunol.* **14**, 481-490.

George, M. and Vaughan, J. H. (1961). *Proc. Soc. exp. Biol. Med.* **111**, 514.

Gershon, R. K. (1974). *In* "Immunological parameters of host-tumour relationships", 198-209 (D. Weiss Ed.) Vol. III. Academic Press, New York and London.

Geswant, W. C., Chasin, L., Tilson, M. D., Rutledge, O. and Goldenberg, I. S. (1971). *Surg. Gynec. Obstet.* **133**, 959-962.

Gold, D. (1967). *Cancer (Philad)* **20**, 1663.

Goldfarb, P. M. and Hardy, M. A. (1975). *Cancer (Philad)* **35**, 778-783.

Goldman, M. (1968). "Fluorescent Antibody Methods". Academic Press, New York and London.

Grace, J. T. (1964). *Ann. N. Y. Acad. Sci.* **114**, 736.

Graham-Pole, J., Ogg, L. J., Ross, C. E. and Cochran, A. J. (1976). *Lancet* **2**, 1376.

Greaves, M. F., Brown, G., Capellard, D., Janossy, G. and Revesz, T. (1976). *In* "Clinical Tumour Immunology" (J. Wybran and M. J. Staquet, Eds.) 115-122. Pergamon Press, Oxford.

Grosser, N. and Thomson, D. M. P. (1975). *Cancer Res.* **35**, 2571-2579.

Gutterman, J. U., Rossen, R. D., Butler, W. T., McCredie, K. B., Bodey, G. P., Freireich, E. J. and Hersh, E. M. (1973). *New Engl. J. Med.* **288**, 169-173.

Halliday, W. J. and Miller, S. (1972). *Int. J. Cancer* **9**, 477.

Halliday, W. J., Maluish, A. E. and Isbister, W. H. (1974). *Brit. J. Cancer* **29**, 31.

Halliday, W. J., Maluish, A. E., Little, J. H. and Davis, N. C. (1975). *Int. J. Cancer* **16**, 645-658.

Hammond, W. G. and Rolley, R. T. (1970). *Cancer (Philad)* **25**, 368-372.

Hardy, W. D., Hess, P. W., MacEwen, G., McLelland, A. J., Zuckerman, E. E., Essex, M., Cotter, S. M. and Jarrett, O. (1976). *Cancer Res.* **36**, 582.

Harrington, J. T. and Stastny, P. (1975). *J. Immunol.* **10**, 752.

Haskill, J. S. and Richmond, M. I. (1973). *J. nat. Cancer Inst.* **51**, 159-163.

Hellström, I. and Sjögren, H. O. (1965). *Exp. Cell Res.* **40**, 212.

Hellström, I., Hellström, K. E., Pierce, G. E. and Bill, A. H. (1968). *Proc. nat. Acad. Sci. (Wash)* **60**, 1231.

Hellström, I. and Hellström, K. E. (1970). *Int. J. Cancer* **5**, 195.

Hellström, I., Hellström, K. E., Bill, A. H., Pierce, G. E. and Yang, J. P. S. (1970). *Int. J. Cancer* **6**, 172.

Hellström, I., Hellström, K. E., Sjögren, H. O. and Warner, G. A. (1971). *Int. J. Cancer* **7**, 1.

Hellström, I., Hellström, K. E., Sjögren, H. O. and Warner, G. A. (1973). *Int. J. Cancer* **11**, 116.

Herschman, H. R. and Lerner, M. P. (1973). *Nature* **241**, 242-244.

Hersey, P., MacLennan, I. C. M., Campbell, A. C., Harris, R. and Freeman, C. B. (1973). *Clin. exp. Immunol.* **14**, 159-167.

Hersh, E. M., Gutterman, J. U., Mavligit, G. M., Granater, C. H., Reed, R. C., Ambus, U. and McBride, C. M. (1975). *Behring Inst. Mitt.* **56**, 139-147.

Hilberg, R. W., Balcerzak, S. P. and Lo Buglio, A. F. (1973). *Cell Immunol.* **7**, 152.

Hólan, V., Hašek, M., Bubeník, J. and Chutná, J. (1974). *Cell Immunol.* **13**, 107-116.

Hollinshead, A. C., Stewart, T. H. M. and Herberman, R. B. (1974). *J. nat. Cancer Inst.* **52**, 327-338.

Hughes, L. E. and Lytton, B. (1964). *Brit. med. J.* **1**, 209.

Humphrey, L., Barker, C. and Bokesch, C. (1971). *Ann. Surg.* **174**, 383-391.

Ikonopisov, R. L., Lewis, M. G., Hunter-Craig, I. D., Bodenham, D. C., Phillips, T. M., Cooling, C. I., Proctor, J., Hamilton Fairley, G. and Alexander, P. (1970). *Brit. med. J.* **2**, 752-754.

Irie, R. F., Irie, K. and Morton, D. L. (1974). *J. nat. Cancer Inst.* **52**, 1051-1057.

Ishizaka, K. (1963). *Progr. Allergy* **7**, 32-106.

Izsak, F. C., Brenner, H. J., Landes, E., Ran, M. and Witz, I. (1974). *Israel J. med. Sci.* **10**, 642.

Johsonn, J., Einhorn, N., Fagraeus, A. and Einhorn, J. (1968). *Radiology.* **90**, 536.

Keisari, Y. and Witz, I. (1975). *Behring Inst. Mitt.* **56**, 19-27.

Klein, G., Sjögren, H. O. and Klein, E. (1962). *Cancer Res.* **22**, 955-961.

Klein, G., Clifford, P., Klein, E., Smith, R. T., Minowada, J., Kourilsky, F. and Burchenal, J. (1967). *J. nat. Cancer Inst.* **39**, 1027.

Kodera, Y. and Bean, M. A. (1975). *Int. J. Cancer* **16**, 579-592.

Kopf, A. W., Silberberg, I. and Cooper, N. S. (1966). *J. invest. Derm.* **47**, 83-86.

Kuhlmann, W. D. and Miller, H. R. P. (1971). *J. Ultrastruct. Res.* **35**, 370-385.

Lampert, F. and Dietmair, E. (1973). *Klin. Woch.* **51**, 198-199.

Leading Article (1976). *Lancet* **1**, 897.

Leneva, N. V. and Svet-Moldavsky, G. J. (1974). *J. nat. Cancer Inst.* **52**, 699-704.

Levin, A. G., McDonough, E. F., Miller, D. G. and Southam, C. M. (1964). *Ann. N.Y. Acad Sci.* **120**, 400.

Levine, P. H., Herberman, R. B., Rosenberg, E. B., McClure, P. D., Roland, A., Pianta, R. J. and Ting, R. C. Y. (1972). *J. nat. Cancer Inst.* **49**, 943-952.

Lewis, M. G., Ikonopisov, R. L., Nairn, R. C., Phillips, T. M., Hamilton Fairley, G., Bodenham, D. C. and Alexander, P. (1969). *Brit. med. J.* **3**, 547.
Lewis, M. G., Phillips, T. M., Cook, K. B. and Blake, J. (1971). *Nature* **232**, 52.
Lewis, M. G., Avis, P. J. G., Phillips, T. M. and Sheikh, K. M. A. (1973). *Yale J. Biol. Med.* **46**, 661-668.
Lewkonia, R. M., Kerr, L. and Irvine, W. J. (1974). *Brit. J. Cancer* **30**, 532-537.
Light, P. A., Preece, E. W. and Waldron, H. A. (1975). *Clin. exp. Immunol.* **22**, 279-284.
Macher, E., Muller, C., Sorg, G., Gassen, A. and Sorg, C. (1975). *Behring Inst. Mitt.* **56**, 86-90.
Mackie, R. M., Spilg, W. G. S., Thomas, C. E., Cameron-Mowat, D. E., Grant, R. M. and Cochran, A. J. (1973). *Rev. de L'Inst. Past. de Lyon* **6**, 281-290.
Maluish, A. E. and Halliday, W. J. (1974). *J. nat. Cancer Inst.* **52**, 1415-1420.
Mancini, G., Carbonara, A. O. and Heremans, J. F. (1965). *Int. J. Immunochem.* **2**, 235-254.
Marti, J. H., Grosser, N. and Thomson, D. M. P. (1976). *Int. J. Cancer* **18**, 48.
Mazuran, R., Mujagic, H., Malenica, B. and Silobrcic, V. (1976). *Int. J. Cancer* **17**, 14.
Möller, E. (1965). *Science* **147**, 873.
Moore, M. and Hughes, L. A. (1973). *Brit. J. Cancer* **28**, Suppl. 1, 175-184.
Morton, D. L. and Malmgren, R. A. (1968). *Science* **162**, 1279.
McGovern, V. J., Mihm, M. C., Bailly, C., Booth, J. C., Clark, W. H., Cochran, A. J., Hardy, E. G., Hicks, J. D., Levene, A., Lewis, M. G., Little, J. H. and Milton, G. W. (1973). *Cancer (Philad)* **32**, 1446-1457.
McLellan, E. (1969). *Brit. J. Surg.* **55**, 850-852.
MacLennan, I. C. M. and Loewi, G. (1968). *Nature* **219**, 1968.
MacLennan, I. C. M., Loewi, G. and Howard, A. (1969). *Immunology* **17**, 887.
MacLennan, I. C. M. (1976). *In* "Clinical Tumour Immunology" (J. Wybran and M. J. Staquet, Eds.) 47-53. Pergamon Press, Oxford.
Nadler, S. H. and Moore, G. E. (1965). *J. Amer. Med. Ass.* **191**, 105-106.
Nairn, R. C., Herzog, F., Ward, H. A. and deBoer, W. G. R. M. (1969). *Clin. exp. Immunol.* **4**, 697.
Nairn, R. C., Nind, A. P. P., Guli, E. P. G., Muller, H. K., Rolland, J. M. and Minty, C. W. (1971a). *Brit. med. J.* **4**, 701-705.
Nairn, R. C., Nind, A. P. P., Guli, E. P. G., Davies, D. J., Rolland, J. M., McGiven, A. R. and Hughes, E. S. R. (1971b). *Brit. med. J.* **4**, 706-709.
Nelson, R. A. (1953). *Science* **118**, 733.
Nishioka, K. (1963a). *J. Immunol.* **90**, 86.
Nishioka, K. and Linscott, W. D. (1963b). *J. exp. Med.* **118**, 767.
Odili, J. L. and Taylor, G. (1971). *Brit. med. J.* **4**, 584-586.
Old, L. J., Boyse, E. A. and Lilly, F. (1963). *Cancer Res.* **23**, 1063-1068.
Oldham, R. K. and Herberman, R. B. (1973). *J. Immunol.* **111**, 1862.
O'Toole, C., Perlmann, P., Unsgaard, B., Moberger, G. and Edsmyr, F. (1972). *Int. J. Cancer* **10**, 77-91.
O'Toole, C., Perlmann, P., Wigzell, H., Unsgaard, B. and Zetterlund, C. G. (1973). *Lancet* **1**, 1085-1088.
Peter, H. H., Diehl, V., Kalden, J. R., Seeland, P. and Eckert, G. (1975). *Behring Inst. Mitt.* **56**, 167.

Pilch, Y. H. and Riggins, R. S. (1966). *Cancer Res.* **26**, 871-875.
Pollack, S., Heppner, G., Brawn, R. J. and Nelson, V. (1972). *Int. J. Cancer* **9**, 316-323.
Porzsolt, F., Tautz, C., Ax, W. (1975). *Behring Inst. Mitt.* **57**, 128.
Powell, A. E., Sloss, A. M., Smith, R. N., Makley, J. T. and Hubay, C. E. (1975). *Int. J. Cancer* **16**, 905-913.
Preece, A. W. and Light, P. A. (1976). *IRCS Med. Sci.* **4**, 201.
Priori, E. S., Wilbur, J. R. and Dmochowski, L. (1971). *J. nat. Cancer Inst.* **46**, 1299-1308.
Pritchard, J. A. V., Moore, J. L., Sutherland, W. H. and Joslin, C. A. F. (1972). *Lancet* **2**, 627-629.
Pross, H. F. and Baines, M. G. (1976). *Int. J. Cancer* **18**, 593-604.
Quismorio, F. P., Bland, S. L. and Friou, G. J. (1971). *Clin. exp. Immunol.* **8**, 701.
Rebuck, J. W. and Crowley, J. H. (1955). *Ann. N.Y. Acad. Sci.* **59**, 757-805.
Rosenberg, E. U., McCoy, J. L., Green, S. S., Donnelly, F. C., Siwarski, D. F., Levine, P. H. and Herberman, R. B. (1974). *J. nat. Cancer Inst.* **52**, 345-352.
Ross, C. E., Cochran, A. J., Jackson, A. M., Mackie, R. M. and Ogg, L. J. (1977). Submitted to *Cancer Immunol. Immunother.*
Sasportes, M., Dehay, C. and Fellous, M. (1971). *Nature* **233**, 332-334.
Scanlon, E. F., Hawkins, R. A., Fox, W. W. and Smith, W. S. (1965). *Cancer (Philad)* **18**, 782-789.
Sega, E., Fegiz, G., Paolini, A., Tosato, F., Casella, M. C. and Citro, G. (1976). *IRCS Med. Sci.* **4**, 106.
Singh, I., Tsang, K. Y. and Blakemore, W. S. (1977). *Nature* **265**, 541.
Skurzak, H. M., Klein, E., Yoshida, T. O. and Lamon, E. W. (1972). *J. exp. Med.* **135**, 997-1002.
Slettenmark, B. and Klein, E. (1962). *Cancer Res.* **22**, 947-954.
Søborg, M. and Bendixen, G. (1967). *Acta med. Scand.* **181**, 247.
Southam, C. M. (1965). *Europ. J. Cancer* **1**, 173.
Spitler, L. E. (1973). *Clin. Res.* **21**, 654.
Stewart, T. H. M. (1969a). *Cancer (Philad)* **23**, 1368-1379.
Stewart, T. H. M. (1969b). *Cancer (Philad)* **23**, 1380-1387.
Stjernswärd, J., Dondal, M., Vánky, F., Wigzell, H. and Sealy, R. (1972). *Lancet* **4**, 1352.
Stonehill, E. H. and Bendich, A. (1970). *Nature* **228**, 370-371.
Sulit, H. S., Golub, S. H., Irie, R., Gupta, R., Grooms, G. A. and Morton, D. L. (1976). *Int. J. Cancer* **17**, 461.
Takasugi, M. and Klein, E. (1970). *Transplant* **9**, 219.
Takasugi, M., Mickey, M. R. and Terasaki, P. I. (1973a). *Nat. Cancer Inst. Monogr.* **37**, 77.
Takasugi, M., Mickey, M. R. and Terasaki, P. I. (1973b). *Cancer Res.* **33**, 2898-2902.
Tautz, C., Khuen, F. and Ax, W. (1974). *Z. Immun-Forsch* **147**, 155-161.
Thunold, S., Tönder, O. and Larsen, O. (1973). *Acta path. microbiol. Scand. A.* (Suppl.) **236**, 97-100.
Vanky, F., Stjernswärd, J., Klein, G. and Nilsonne, U. (1971). *J. nat. Cancer Inst.* **47**, 95-103.
Vanky, F., Klein, E., Stjernswärd, J. and Nilsonne, U. (1974). *Int. J. Cancer* **14**, 277.
Vanky, F., Klein, E. and Stjernswärd, J. (1976). In "Clinical Tumour Immunology" (J. Wybran and M. J. Staquet, Eds.) 55-68. Pergamon Press, Oxford.
Vianna, N. J., Greenwald, P. and Davies, J. N. P. (1971). *Lancet* **1**, 1209.

Whitehouse, J. M. A. (1973). *Brit. J. Cancer* **28** Suppl. 1, 170-174.
Winters, W. D. and Morton, D. L. (1973). "Host environment interactions in the Etiology of Cancer in Man" (R. Doll and I. Vodopija, Eds.) 331-335. (IARC, Lyon. Scientific Publications No. 7).
Witz, I., Klein, G. and Pressman, D. (1969). *Proc. Soc. exp. Biol. Med.* **130,** 1102. (1969). *Proc. Soc. exp. Biol. Med.* **130,** 1102.
Witz, I. and Ran, M. (1970). *In* "Immunity and Tolerance in Oncogenesis" (L. Severi Ed.) 345-354. University of Perugia, Italy.

4

Antigens on Tumour Cells

The tumour cell, like other cells is bounded by a complex bilipid membrane which is traversed by glycoprotein molecules which protrude from the surface for varying lengths.

The immunodominant prosthetic groups are mainly carbohydrate molecules which by their complexity and pliancy under the influence of electrostatic and hydrophobic forces permit much greater polymorphism than the same number of protein or lipid molecules. The cell surface is thus a forest of molecular stumps which serve a variety of functions such as maintenance of structure, the reception, fixation and enzymic modification of metabolic molecules prior to their transport into the cell, cellular recognition (possibly by identification of the profiles of Ig-like molecules), cell-cell union in the case of squamous epithelia and the export of secretion products from glandular epithelia.

In a normal adult cell the stereogeometry of surface molecules and that of the various combinations of neighbouring molecules is recognisable as self and does not initiate an auto-immune response. However, the development of absolutely new molecules, or a drastic modification of existing molecular structure or deletion of molecules, causing alteration of the profile of adjacent molecules or unmasking of normally covered molecules may create a non-self stimulus (Fig. 4.1). If this is sufficiently strong an "auto-immune" reaction, against only slightly modified self, will result. It is against such evolution of membrane characteristics that the lymphoid system is claimed to act in immune surveillance. Operationally any new or modified molecule which renders a cell auto-immunogenic may be regarded as a "neo-antigen", regardless of whether the change results from an endogenous alteration of cellular activities or changes imposed by extraneously derived factors such as viruses or chemicals.

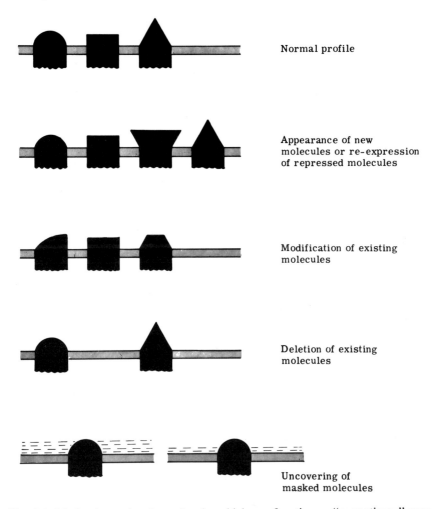

Normal profile

Appearance of new
molecules or re-expression
of repressed molecules

Modification of existing
molecules

Deletion of existing
molecules

Uncovering of
masked molecules

Fig. 4.1. Mechanisms whereby molecules which can function as "neoantigens" may
appear on cell membranes and render the cell autoimmunogenic.

A further source of potentially immunogenic molecules is the interior of
the cell. Such molecules may derive from the cytoplasm, intracellular
organelles or the nucleus and nucleoli and are released to the extracellular
environment during secretion and after cell breakdown. The absence of
antibodies to such components in a majority of the general population
suggests that they are not normally immunogenic. This may be due to
enzymic degradation or masking of determinant sites, or to self tolerance or
because the amounts released at any one time are very small. The possible

importance of tolerance is supported by the progressive increase in auto-antibodies seen in ageing populations. That intracellular molecules can be immunogenic is shown by the development of autoantibodies to them in autoimmune disease, for instance antimicrosomal antibodies in autoimmune thyroiditis.

Anticytoplasmic, antinuclear and antinucleolar antibodies have also been found in cancer patients. It is not clear, however, whether such antibodies influence the clinical progression of cancer or are merely a result of the release of intracellular molecules (after tumour necrosis) in a quantity and form able to trigger an immune response or break tolerance. Antibodies to cytoplasmic components certainly are maximal late in the disease. It is, in fact difficult to see how antibodies to intracellular components could affect the survival, replication or mobility of intact tumour cells. Antibodies to membrane-located components seem better suited to such tumour-inhibitory roles. This does not, however, exclude an immunosuppressive or effector cell blocking activity for intracellular antigens complexed to the appropriate antibodies.

Membrane Characteristics of Tumour Cells

Despite their remarkable characteristics of local spread and metastasis tumour cells share many structural, biochemical and functional charac-teristics of normal cells, including common cell membrane characteristics. However tumour cells possess features absent from comparable mature normal cells, or present at low frequency on such cells.

SPECIES MARKERS

Tumour cells bear this type of molecule at about the same frequency as normal cells. When attempts are made to raise xenogeneic antisera to tumour cells, extensive absorption is always necessary to remove anti-species antibodies. Tumour transplantation from species to species is not generally feasible in intact animals, but is possible if the tumour is placed in an immunologically privileged site, such as the anterior chamber of the eye (Green, 1950) the hamster cheek pouch (Richmond and Morton, 1974) or guinea pig cerebrum (Manuelidis, 1971) or in animals which are congenitally athymic (Povlsen and Rygaard, 1971; Giovanella et al., 1972) or deliberately made immunodeficient. This has most often been achieved by treatment with antithymocyte serum (Detre and Gazet, 1973) or irradiation and thymectomy followed by bone marrow cell reconstitution (Castro, 1972; Franks et al., 1973). Human tumours grow and metastasise in such xenogeneic hosts and provide an excellent opportunity for studying the effect of immunological factors in vivo and the effectiveness of different therapeutic agents.

TRANSPLANTATION ANTIGENS

Mainly as a result of increased interest in organ allografting, much is now known about the genetic control and biochemistry of these markers of individuality in man. They are present on tumour cells at a frequency similar to that on normal cells, although cancer sera may contain factors capable of masking specific antigens (Clark *et al.*, 1974). Failure to appreciate the existence of transplantation antigen disparities was a major reason for the failure of early attempts to study the tumour immunology of outbred laboratory animals. There have been numerous studies of the HL-A type of patients with a variety of cancers in an attempt to identify individuals with special susceptibility. Such associations have been reported (Chapter 2) but it is not known how HL-A type predisposes to a cancer and in particular whether the actual molecular configuration of the transplantation antigens at the cell membrane is important. Recent studies indicate association between genes coding for transplantation antigens and some genes controlling immune responsiveness (Benacerraf and McDevitt, 1972) and it has to be established whether it is this or some other association which is crucial rather than the actual identity of the transplantation antigens. Choriocarcinoma presents a special situation, being a half-allograft. There are claims that the probability of development of a trophoblastic tumour is related to histocompatibility differences between the patient and the male partner in the conception (Morgenson *et al.*, 1969; Ivaskova *et al.*, 1969) and that maternal-paternal HL-A antigen disparity protects against dissemination of choriocarcinoma (Morgenson *et al.*, 1969). This view is not universally shared but the observations indicate important areas for study.

BLOOD GROUP ANTIGENS

These too are present on many different cells including certain tumour cells. However on some tumour cells their frequency is reduced relative to that on normal cells.

ORGAN-SPECIFIC MARKERS

These are widely distributed on tumour cells and normal cells, although a decline in their frequency has been reported in some cancer cells (Goudie and McCallum, 1963).

Human tumours of similar histogenesis share cross reacting antigens which raises the possibility that some of these antigens may be of organ-specific type. In a study of breast tissue extracts, cancer patients' leucocytes reacted selectively to extracts of breast cancer, but did not react with extracts of normal breast tissue any more frequently than did leucocytes from normal individuals or from patients with non-cancerous breast disease. Normal leucocytes and those from patients with non-cancerous breast disease seldom reacted with extracts of breast cancer (Cochran *et al.*, 1974, and Table 4.1). McCoy *et al.* (1974) found a similar situation. These findings suggest that the antigens detected are tumour related or that if they are organ-specific they are less numerous on normal cells or present in a modified and less immunogenic form.

Table 4.1.

The effect of extracts of cancerous and non-cancerous breast tissues on the migration of leucocytes from patients with various breast conditions and normal donors. (Cochran *et al.*, 1974.)

Leucocyte donor	Tissue extract		
	Breast cancer	Simple breast disease	Normal breast
Breast cancer	97/138[a] (70)	4/19 (21)	3/13 (23)
Simple breast disease	18/96 (19)	1/6 (17)	2/9 (22)
Normal people	9/33 (27)	1/6 (17)	

[a] No. of positive reactors/Total of individuals tested (%).

ONCOFOETAL ANTIGENS

Attention has recently been centred on the observation that some antigens which are detectable at relatively high concentration on tumour cells are molecules which are normally synthesised only by the appropriate precursor cells during certain stages of embryogenesis. These antigens are either completely absent from normal adult cells, or more probably are present at very low concentration. In malignant cells, therefore, genes which are normally repressed are permitted to function, an event which accords well with the tendency of tumour cells to possess more primitive or embryonic characteristics.

An increasing number of oncofoetal (OF) antigens has been recognised and a selection of such molecules is shown in Table 4.2. Even from this short list the diversity of tumours bearing OF antigens is clear. It seems likely that with increasing investigation this type of molecule will be found on all, or virtually all, types of human tumour cells. This has certainly been found to be the case in adequately studied animal systems where, however, the co-existence of carcinogen-related neoantigens is common. Thus the observation of OF antigens on human tumour cells is no excuse for abandoning the search for other molecules which may reflect carcinogenesis or the processes of malignant transformation.

It is appropriate to consider two of the best known human OF antigens in more detail.

Table 4.2.

A selection of oncofoetal antigens

Antigen	Tumour	Reference
Intestinal antigen	Increased gastric cancer	Nairn et al. (1962). Brit. med. J. **1**, 1791
α-fetoprotein	Mouse hepatoma	Abelev et al. (1963). Transplant **1**, 174
α-fetoprotein	Human hepatoma	Tatarinov, J. S. (1964). Vop. Med. Khim. **10**, 90
Carcinoembryonic antigen	Endodermal and other tumours	Gold and Freedman (1965). J. Exp. Med. **121**, 439
Foetal sulfoglycoprotein	Gastric cancer	Hakkinen et al. (1968). Int. J. Cancer **3**, 572
Gastric antigen	Decreased gastric ulcer	deBoer et al. (1969). Brit. med. J. J. **3**, 93
α₂H globulin	Childhood tumours	Buffe et al. (1970). Int. J. Cancer **5**, 85
Foetal antigens	Gliomas	Gold, P. A. (1971). Rev. Med. **22**, 85
γ FP antigen	Various	Edynak et al. (1972). New Engl. J. Med. **286**, 1178
Carcinofoetal ferritin	Hepatomas	Alpert et al. (1973). Nature **242**, 194
Foetal antigens	Melanoma	Avis and Lewis (1973). J. nat. Cancer Inst. **51**, 1063
Foetal antigens	Leukaemia	Baker and Taub (1973). Nature (New Biol.) **241**, 93
Foetal antigens	Hodgkin's disease	Katz et al. (1973). Proc. nat. Acad. Sci. **70**, 396
S2 antigen	Sarcomas	Mukherji and Hirshaut (1973). Science **181**, 440
Foetal antigens	Melanomas	Macher et al. (1975). Behring Inst. Mitt. **56**, 86
Foetal antigens	Melanomas	Hersey et al. (1977). Int. J. Cancer **18**, 564

Alpha-fetoprotein (α-FP)

This α globulin was identified in the serum of mouse embryos and in mouse hepatomas by Abelev (1963) and subsequently in human hepatomas by Tatarinov (1964). Significantly, levels of circulating α-FP were only slightly raised in most patients with secondary cancer in the liver (Ruoslahti et al., 1972). However markedly raised levels have been recorded in germ cell tumours such as ovarian and testicular teratomas (Alpert et al., 1971; Smith and O'Neill, 1971). In hepatoma patients the detection rate initially varied with the ethnic background and the test employed (Abelev, 1971), however, more sensitive tests such as radioimmunoassay have increased the detection rate (Thomson *et al.*, 1973). The price for this is increased detection of α-FP in non-hepatoma situations with consequent difficulties of interpretation.

Carcinoembryonic antigen (CEA)

This highly branched glycoprotein (mol. wt 200 000) was described by Gold and Freedman (1965) as occurring in human colon cancer and in foetal gut, pancreas and liver up to the sixth month of gestation. It was initially held that CEA was absent from normal adult endodermal tissues and tumours other than colon carcinoma, but the use of increasingly sensitive tests has shown it to be very widely distributed in normal tissues and cancers of many different organs (Reynoso *et al.*, 1972). There are probably at least six molecular species of CEA (Everleigh, 1972). Increased levels have also been recorded in a variety of inflammatory conditions and its association with growth and reparative activities has led to the suggestion that CEA may be functionally involved in such processes. The role of CEA in diagnosis, monitoring and prognostication will be considered in Chapter 7.

We do not know whether OF antigens are merely epiphenomena or have a significant rôle in tumour evolution. In animals immunity to embryonal antigens modifies the fate of tumour grafts (for review see Coggin and Anderson, 1974) and immunisation against tumours reduces the growth of embryo tissue implants (Salinas *et al.*, 1972) and may reduce the size of subsequent litters or of individual foetuses (Parmiani and Della Porta, 1973). Lymph node cells from pregnant animals inhibit the growth of tumour cells *in vitro*, which activity may be abrogated by extracts of foetal cells (Brawn, 1970) and sera from multiparous animals (Coggin and Anderson, 1974). In human studies it was found that pregnant and menopausal women had antibodies which reacted with apparently foetal antigens on melanoma cells (Hersey *et al.*, 1977b). Women who had previously been pregnant survived longer and had a lower incidence of dissemination than men, and women who had not been pregnant despite a similar incidence of primary melanoma (Hersey *et al.*, 1977a).

While these observations indicate a possible positive role for immune responses to expressed foetal antigens in tumour rejection or containment it has to be considered whether they may also have a deleterious effect. Transiently expressed auto-antigenic molecules may protect the developing foetus by acting as tolerogens or by blocking potentially damaging lymphoid cells by release of free antigen, the formation of immune complexes or the induction of non-cytotoxic antibodies which coat cells bearing the appropriate antigens. The more fixed expression of these same antigens on tumour cells may alter the nature of any resulting immune response and a major blocking effect which might overwhelm any rejection inducing activities of other tumour-associated antigens seems possible.

Other alterations in keeping with the reversion of tumour cells to a more primitive state include the development of placental antigens (Tal *et al.*, 1964) and hormones in patients with non-trophoblastic malignancies (Weintraub and Rosen, 1971), the synthesis of tumour angiogenesis factor (Greenblatt and Shubik, 1968), the recurrence of foetal forms of haemoglobin (Singer *et al.*, 1951; Miller, 1969) and of foetal enzymes (Criss, 1971) such as the heat-stable alkaline phosphatase known as the Regan Isoenzyme (Fishman *et al.*, 1968). The "inappropriate" production of hormones by non-endocrine tumours may also be interpreted as a reversionary change.

CARCINOGEN ASSOCIATED ANTIGENS

These have been extensively studied in animals where the carcinogen employed is known, the experimental conditions can be controlled and the kinetics of cell membrane alteration followed closely. The general finding has been that new membrane-located antigens do appear *pari passu* with malignant transformation and are products of modification of the cell genome by the carcinogen and consequently altered cellular biosynthetic mechanisms. However, the immunogenic "strength" of the antigens varies with the type of carcinogen employed, its dose and route of administration and the species tested.

Tumours induced by the same virus share antigens which relate to the inducing virus (Klein *et al.*, 1960; Habel, 1961). This is true of tumours arising in different members of the same strain, members of different strains and even in members of different species. Chemical carcinogen induced tumours on the other hand possess unique antigens which do not show identity or similarity in attempted cross reactivity or cross protection studies. (Old *et al.*, 1962; Baldwin and Barker, 1967). This was found even where two tumours were induced by the same chemical. Tumours induced by physical agents, such as radiant energy or plastic films also have predominantly non-cross reacting antigens. The above probably oversimplifies the situation and some reports have claimed that there may be minor individual unique antigens on virus induced tumours and that some chemically-induced tumours may have weak shared antigens additional to the dominant unique antigens (Prehn and Main, 1957; Globerson and Feldman, 1964). "Spontaneous" tumours are spontaneous only in the sense that we are ignorant of the carcinogenic mechanisms involved. Most tumours of this type in animals possess distinctly weak and relatively unique antigens, although by definition it is difficult to ascertain their degree of exclusiveness.

Despite the above noted qualifications the important general principle of the shared antigenicity of viral tumours and the individuality of the antigens of chemical tumours holds true in an operational sense. This is critical as cross protection by immunological means and immunoprophylaxis are possible if tumours share antigens, as has been shown in a multitude of animal studies. Protection by immunisation is clearly not possible for tumours which lack common membrane antigens.

This dilemma provides excellent justification for continuing attempts to ascertain whether at least some human tumours are virus induced. Reports of cross reacting antigens on human tumours of identical histogenesis may be interpreted as favouring viral involvement in their aetiology. The situation cannot, however, be accepted without a consideration of alternative explanations. I have already discussed the possibility that some of these antigens may be organ specific or oncofoetal in nature. Another interpretation, which is almost impossible to disprove, is that transformed or transforming cells are specially susceptible to virus infection and that while the membrane-located neoantigens *are* virus-determined the virus is merely a passenger and has little or nothing to do with initiation of malignant transformation. The cross reactive similarity of the antigens detected on human tumours of similar histogenesis is against this thesis. If the susceptibility to passenger virus hypothesis were true, the findings would imply susceptibility restricted to only a very few viruses, which is unproved and seems unlikely. Further, as yet unproven, possibilities are that during the processes of malignant transformation latent viruses within the cell are activated or virogenes (viral materials integrated in the genome) are derepressed and induce the observed membrane changes.

We do not know the carcinogen(s) responsible for most human tumours, which effectively prevents the identification of neoantigens as carcinogen-associated in man. The nearest approach to this is in tumours in which observational and circumstantial evidence favour the involvement of a virus in their aetiology. The main tumour to be considered is Burkitt lymphoma (BL) which has been meticulously examined from many different standpoints during the past fifteen years. These studies of BL serve as a model against which investigations of other tumours must stand comparison. Although it is clearly impossible to undertake tumour transplantation or virus transfer in a human situation, the weight of evidence increasingly favours viral complicity in the aetiology of BL. Viral oncogenesis has also been considered in other tumours such as nasopharyngeal carcinoma, Hodgkin's disease, breast cancer in women, carcinoma of the cervix uteri and acute leukaemia, however the evidence for viral participation in the causation of these tumours is markedly weaker than is the case with BL.

Burkitt lymphoma (BL)

This is a malignant B cell lymphoma which is relatively common in areas of defined geographical and climatological characteristics in Africa and New

Guinea but also occurs sporadically throughout the rest of the world where the incidence has been calculated as one hundredth that of the high incidence areas. It mainly affects the facial and abdominal tissues of children. On the basis of the restricted characteristics of the areas of high incidence, time-space clustering of cases and seasonal variation of case incidence viral involvement in carcinogenesis has been considered possible (Burkitt, 1963; Morrow *et al.*, 1976). Studies of suspension cultures of BL by immunofluorescence (IF) showed antibodies to cytoplasmic and membrane components in sera from BL patients (Henle and Henle, 1966; Henle *et al.*, 1969). The frequency of IF positive cells correlated with the presence within them of particles of a virus described by Epstein *et al.* (1964) and subsequently identified as a new member of the herpes virus group, now known as Epstein-Barr virus (EBV) and the cause of Paul-Bunnell positive infectious mononucleosis (Henle *et al.*, 1968; Niederman *et al.*, 1968). Antibodies to EBV related antigens were found to occur in 90% of adults in the general population of Western countries, but the age at which antibodies to EBV developed varied from population to population and the titre of antibodies detected never approached that which has come to be regarded as the *sine qua non* of BL. EBV infection can induce up to five virus-related new antigens which vary in the timing of their development after primary infection and in their biological significance. These are membrane antigen (MA), viral capsid antigen (VCA), early antigen (EA), Epstein Barr virus nuclear antigen (EBNA) and lymphocyte determined membrane antigen (LYDMA). The vast majority of human B lymphocyte cell lines carry EBV DNA and express EBNA and LYDMA which are markers of the presence of EBV DNA. The presence of MA, EA and VCA indicates that the virus-cell interaction will eventually lead to cell lysis. The detection of these antigens and antibodies to them is obviously of diagnostic importance in appropriate clinical situations. That the virus has an aetiological role is strongly favoured by the constant presence of EBV DNA in BL cells, the strength and consistency of the immunological reaction to the virus determined antigens, the capacity of EBV to transform human lymphocytes *in vitro* (Henle *et al.*, 1967; Pope *et al.*, 1968) and its ability to induce lymphomas in higher primates (Epstein *et al.*, 1973). However the ubiquity of antibodies to EBV in the general population suggests that EBV exposure leads to a subclinical infection or the syndrome of infectious mononucleosis in the majority of individuals, the outcome being determined by factors such as genetic constitution, age and physical condition at the time of infection. At present, we cannot exclude the possibility that there are several strains of EBV which might have different patterns of pathogenicity. For EBV infection to result in BL other cofactors such as chronic reticuloendothelial stimulation by holoendemic malaria may require to be operative. The situation is further complicated by recent suggestions that "C"-type viruses may have a helper role (Kufe *et al.*, 1973).

Raised titres of antibodies to EBV have also been reported in patients with other tumours, such as nasopharyngeal carcinoma (NPC) (deSchryver *et al.*, 1969), acute lymphoblastic leukaemia (Levine *et al.*, 1972a), chronic lymphocytic leukaemia and lymphocytic lymphoma (Johansson *et al.*, 1971), chronic lymphocytic and chronic myeloid leukaemia (Levine *et al.*, 1972b) and Hodgkin's disease (Levine *et al.*, 1970; Johansson *et al.*, 1970). The case for an aetiological role in NPC is relatively strong, that for the other malignancies is less so, and the altered reaction to EBV may be a result of disturbances of general immunity known to occur in Hodgkin's disease and the leukaemias.

Breast cancer (BC)
Tumour directed cellular immunity (Andersen *et al.*, 1970; Cochran *et al.*, 1972; Segall *et al.*, 1972; Black *et al.*, 1974a; McCoy *et al.*, 1974) and humoral immunity (Priori *et al.*, 1971; Edynak *et al.*, 1972) have been demonstrated in women with breast cancer. Distinctive proteins have been extracted from breast cancers (Hollinshead *et al.*, 1974; Black *et al.*, 1976) and induce skin reactions in women with breast carcinoma.

Black and his colleagues have extended these observations and report that the anti-tumour immune reaction in BC cross reacts with antigens on mouse mammary tumour virus (MTV) (Black *et al.*, 1974b). This observation accords with previous findings suggestive of an association between human BC and MTV. "B"-type virus particles identical in ultrastructural morphology to those seen in mouse mammary cancer have been seen in human breast cancers and in the milk of women with breast cancer and such milk may neutralise MTV as can factors in the serum of women with BC (Dmochowski and Bowen, 1973). Schlom and Spiegelman (1973) reported that RNA from some breast cancers could be hybridised with DNA made by reverse transcriptase on an MTV RNA template, although others have found this to be uncommon (Vaidya *et al.*, 1974). The situation remains to be finally established but it seems probable that antigens related to MTV or a closely similar agent appear on the membranes of the cells of at least some breast cancers. The aetiological significance of this is unknown.

Carcinoma of the cervix uteri
Relative to age matched controls women with cervical dysplasia, carcinoma-in-situ or invasive squamous carcinoma have a raised incidence of cell-mediated immunity to herpes simplex virus, type 2 (HSV-2), neutralising antibodies to HSV-2, and antibodies to various structural and non-virion antigens of HSV-2 (Aurelian and Strnad, 1976). Structural antigens and non-virion antigens are detectable on exfoliated tumour cells and on the cells

comprising tumours. HSV-2 has been isolated from a culture of carcinoma-in-situ and a small proportion of cultured tumour cells, though not producing virus, bear HSV-2 membrane antigens (Aurelian, 1974; Aurelian *et al.*, 1971). By contrast HSV-2 DNA has been identified in cervical carcinoma cells only once (Frenkel *et al.*, 1972). HSV-2 can transform human embryo cells (Takahashi and Yamanishi, 1974) and induces dysplastic cervical changes in Cebus monkeys (Palmer *et al.*, 1976). There is thus a clear association between Herpes simplex virus, type 2 and carcinoma of the cervix uteri but an aetiological relationship remains unproven.

OTHER CHANGES IN CHARACTERISTICS OF TUMOUR CELL MEMBRANES

The undernoted membrane characteristics represent further differences between the molecular constitution of tumour cells and normal cells. They are not necessarily associated with auto-immunogenicity, but are included because they seem likely to contribute to our understanding of the host-tumour interaction.

Lectin binding and cell agglutinability

Lectins are plant extracts which, by binding to specific membrane located carbohydrate molecules, may cause agglutination of cells. Tumour cells and embryonal cells are more readily agglutinated by lectins than are normal cells. However, treatment of normal cells with proteolytic enzymes renders them as agglutinable as tumour cells, suggesting that the majority of lectin binding sites on normal cells are usually masked. There is variation in lectin binding site exposure at different stages of the cell cycle and the altered situation in tumour cells and embryonal cells may merely reflect their particular cell-cycle characteristics (see Rapin and Burger, 1974 for review).

Receptors for the Fc portion of immunoglobulin

Receptors for the Fc portion of immunoglobulin have been demonstrated on the surface of cells in a variety of benign and malignant tumours in animals (Milgrom *et al.*, 1968; Cohen *et al.*, 1971) and man (Thunold *et al.*, 1970; Tønder and Thunold, 1973; Tønder *et al.*, 1975). The function of these receptors is unknown, but, if they are truly on tumour cells and not on infiltrating macrophages of lymphocytes, by binding immunoglobulin molecules they may coat the cell membrane and exclude effector cells, causing in this way a non-specific blocking effect. The Fc receptor concentration varies from tumour to tumour and it has been suggested that this may form the basis of a new method of classification. Wide variations in receptor frequency from cell to cell within tumours make this possibility somewhat less attractive.

Tumour antigens detectable by inoculation into animals

Predictably, animals injected with human tumour tissue respond by mounting an immune response. Numerous attempts have been made to exploit this to produce materials for the study of tumour associated antigens, for immuno-diagnosis and for immunotherapy. The major problem is that the animals react to many different immunogens, including species markers, serum proteins, blood group antigens and transplantation antigens as well as tumour-associated antigens (TAA); the TAA being generally weakly immunogenic relative to the other groups of antigens, any immune response raised against tumour tissue is inevitably polyspecific, and to render it tumour specific is technically demanding.

The majority of studies have sought to raise antisera to TAA (Hirszfeld *et al.*, 1929; Witebsky, 1930; Metzgar *et al.*, 1973; Bell and Seetharam, 1976) and most authors record considerable difficulty in the extensive absorption phase necessary to remove activities to antigens other than TAA from what Milgrom (1961) aptly called a "jungle of serological reactions". Removal of such "extraneous" activity was often associated with complete or near complete removal of anti-tumour activity. Nonetheless, carefully controlled studies of appropriately absorbed antisera have demonstrated TAA on a variety of tumour cells (Bell and Seetharam, 1976; Metzgar *et al.*, 1972; Harris *et al.*, 1971; Mahn *et al.*, 1972; Halterman *et al.*, 1973).

An even more complex approach has been to sensitise animals to *tumour* materials, desensitise them by exposure to appropriate *normal* tissues and subsequently challenge them with tissues bearing the putative TAA. TAA are detected by observing an immune reaction in the sensitised animals on challenge with the appropriate tumour tissues but not with control tissues. The intact animal may be used and a systemic anaphylactic reaction taken as the end-point, or isolated tissues such as gut or uterus used *in vitro* to detect anaphylaxis or Schultz-Dale type reactions (see Zilber and Abelev, 1968; Makari, 1958; Burrows, 1958; Grace and Lehoczky, 1959; Hackett and Gardonyi, 1960). This approach, while theoretically attractive, involves considerable time and expertise in preparation of animals and is now largely superseded by sophisticated biochemical preparative techniques and the *in vitro* immunological techniques discussed above.

ISOLATION AND PURIFICATION OF TUMOUR ASSOCIATED ANTIGENS

There is considerable interest in the possibility of extracting individual antigens from tumour cell membranes. Purified antigens offer the possibility of identification of their composition and structure and should permit greatly increased specificity in studies of tumour immunity *in vivo* and *in vitro* and the development of radioimmunoassays. It might also be possible eventually to synthesise the antigens and employ them in immunodiagnosis and active specific immunotherapy. The main approach is to extract antigens by disrupting the cell membrane physically, enzymatically or by exposure to hypertonic solutions such as 3M KCl. The resulting separated membrane components are further purified by techniques such as column chromatography, differential centrifugation, filtration, dialysis and electrophoresis. The fractions obtained from tumour cells are compared with those from relevant normal adult and foetal tissues and those unique to the tumour identified and harvested for further study. The extent of the necessary preparative techniques and the dislocation of the antigens from adjacent molecules raises the possibility that the final product may not truly reflect the immunogenic molecule as seen by the recognition cells of the immune system *in vivo*. However, the specificity of reactions observed with these preparations suggests that this theoretical problem is not encountered in practice. These techniques have been used in studies of various tumours including melanoma (Hollinshead *et al.*, 1974b; Char *et al.*, 1974; Roth *et al.*, 1976) gastric cancer (Hollinshead and Herberman, 1973) and lung cancer (Hollinshead *et al.*, 1974c; Hollinshead and Stewart, 1977). Several tumour associated antigens have been identified on the tumours studied and, while some have been identified as re-expressed foetal antigens or related to Herpes simplex virus (lung cancer—Hollinshead and Stewart, 1977) others at present seem tumour specific. An important observation is that there exist materials on tumour cells which can inhibit cell mediated immunity *in vivo* and *in vitro*, which goes some way to explaining the low frequency of reactions induced by crude membrane extracts (Hollinshead and Herberman, 1973; Roth *et al.*, 1976). Electrophoresis purified lung cancer membrane antigens are currently employed in a trial of active specific immunotherapy (Hollinshead and Stewart, 1977).

SHEDDING OF MEMBRANE ANTIGENS

Tumour cells release plasma membrane components, including tumour associated antigens into the body fluids at a rate which varies from tumour to tumour (Currie and Basham, 1972; Baldwin *et al.*, 1973; Currie and Alexander, 1974). It has been suggested that the tumours which most readily shed antigens are those most able to metastasise. Released TAA may act as a "smoke screen", the free antigens combining directly with specific receptor sites of sensitised lymphocytes and blocking them or with anti-tumour antibodies forming immune complexes which may also block effector cells (Chapter 5). It is of interest that antigen shedding has been considered as one mechanism of self tolerance (Cohen *et al.*, 1974).

Variations in Antigen Expression on Cells During the Process of Tumour Development

The extent to which TAA are unique to tumour cells remains of central importance in tumour immunology. Oncofoetal antigens, while maximally expressed on tumour cells and the cells of the embryo (often during a relatively restricted period) are probably also present, though at low concentration on normal adult cells. Newly acquired TAA, such as those induced by oncogenic agents would be expected to be absent from truly normal cells. The expression of such antigens on the cells of simple tumours and on cells undergoing hyperplasia, dysplasia or involved in the *in situ* phase of malignancy has however been relatively little studied, although from a basic scientific point of view and for practical reasons, such information would be of considerable value. If TAA are expressed on the cells of *in situ* malignancy and are shed into body fluids their detection and the demonstration of increasing quantities in serial tests would provide a useful screening assay for early cancer.

Indirect evidence for altered tissue immunogenicity is provided by morphological studies which show infiltrates of lymphoreticular cells in the absence of any other antigenic stimulus (Chapter 2). While exceptions do exist, it is generally true that simple tumours do not attract this type of infiltrate while premalignant conditions and *in situ* malignancy are usually attended by "inflammatory" infiltrates.

Limited laboratory studies of simple tumours and premalignant tissues have been undertaken and suggest that neoantigens exist on tumours early in carcinogenesis and in precancer (Prehn and Slemmer, 1967; Lappé, 1968; Turk, 1969), in tissues exposed to doses of carcinogen insufficient to produce malignancy and in tumours which eventually regress, such as the Shope papilloma (Hellström *et al.*, 1969). A similar situation is suggested in man by studies of leukoplakia (Lehner, 1970) keratoacanthoma (Brown and Tan, 1973), breast disease and melanocytic anomalies (see below).

MELANOCYTE ANOMALIES AND TUMOURS

The tumours and growth aberrations of melanocytes provide an excellent model. Tissue, lymphocytes and serum can be obtained from individuals with simple melanocytic hyperplasia (Lentigenes, lentigo simplex), simple melanocytic tumours (intradermal and compound naevi), *malignant melanoma in situ* (lentigo maligna, superficial spreading melanoma *in situ*) and invasive malignant melanoma. These tissues may be analysed for evidence of neoantigenicity and peripheral blood leucocytes from individuals with these conditions examined for evidence of sensitisation to antigens on the cells of the various normal, hyperplastic, preneoplastic and overtly neoplastic tissues.

The main deficiency of this model is that it has not proved possible to obtain pure preparations of normal melanocytes to examine their antigenicity. Culture of melanocytes is possible, but does not yield sufficiently large numbers of cells for study purposes, and in any case such cells are less than ideal as none of the other cells examined are tissue culture derived. The ingenious use of normal choroidal melanocytes in studies of anti-tumour antibodies in ocular melanoma described by Federman et al. (1976) is not applicable to studies of skin melanoma and the provision of sufficient cells presents probably insuperable logistic problems. The best source of "normal" melanocyte antigens appears to be extracts of histologically normal skin although there is inevitably a low concentration of melanocyte-derived antigens relative to those derived from keratinocytes in this type of preparation.

From table 4.3 it may be seen that naevus patients' leucocytes* were infrequently reactive with naevus extracts and at a frequency no higher than that of normal individuals' leucocytes while melanoma patients' leucocytes reacted with naevus extracts more frequently than those of normal donors (p <0·02) and naevus patients (p <0·02). Two conclusions may be drawn from these findings. First, patients with benign melanocytic tumours are seldom spontaneously sensitised to their own tumours or the tumours of others of similar histogenesis. Second, the limited preferential reactivity of melanoma leucocytes with naevus preparations suggests that antigens with at least structural similarity to melanoma associated antigens are present on naevi, probably at a lower concentration than on melanoma cells, necessitating the strongly sensitised lymphocytes of melanoma patients to detect them. However in a comparable, but smaller study, McCoy et al. (1975) found melanoma leucocytes non-reactive with a 3M KC1 extract of a

Table 4.3.

The reaction of leucocytes from normal individuals, patients with simple naevi and patients with malignant melanoma with extracts of simple naevi and malignant melanoma in the leucocyte migration test. (Wilson et al., In Press.)

Leucocyte donors	Extract from			
	Simple naevi		Malignant melanoma	
	+/T[a]	(%)	+/T	(%)
Normal donors	14/98	(14)	9/64	(14)
Naevus patients	6/52	(12)	9/23	(39)
Melanoma patients	16/51	(31)	34/56	(61)

[a]Individuals positive/total individuals tested.

*We all have naevi! In this context patients are individuals presenting at a dermatology clinic with a history of change in a naevus; growth, altered pigmentation or ulceration.

naevus. Naevus patients' leucocytes reacted more frequently with melanoma extracts than did normal leucocytes (p <0·01) indicating that a proportion of naevus patients are sensitised to antigens cross reactive with melanoma-associated antigens.

Since melanoma patients' lymphocytes provide a sensitive probe for melanoma associated antigens we examined their reactivity with extracts of normal skin, skin from areas around melanomas where there was melanocyte pleomorphism and hyperplasia and skin from areas of lentigo maligna (Table 4.4). Preferential reactivity of melanoma patients' leucocytes with extracts of peritumoral skin and lentigo maligna but no selective activity with normal skin suggests that neoantigenicity is associated with pleomorphism and *in situ* malignant change of melanocytes.

Table 4.4.

The reaction of leucocytes from normal individuals, naevus patients and melanoma patients with extracts of normal skin, peritumoral skin and lentigo maligna in the leucocyte migration test. (Wilson *et al.*, In Press.)

	Extract from					
Leucocyte donors	Normal skin		Peritumoral skin		Lentigo maligna	
	+/T[a]	(%)	+/T	(%)	+/T	(%)
Normal donors	2/24	(8)	2/31	(7)	5/23	(22)
Naevus patients	0/18	(0)	8/30	(27)	5/17	(29)
Melanoma patients	5/19	(26)	28/44	(64)	20/35	(57)

[a]Individuals positive/total individuals tested.

Sutton's halo naevus (Fig. 2.3) a pigmented cutaneous lesion which undergoes regressive changes in association with the formation of an area of depigmentation around it has generated considerable recent interest. Histological examination shows changes which vary with the timing of the biopsy relative to the regression. The basic appearances are of a melanocytic lesion infiltrated by lymphoid cells and macrophages, tumour cell destruction and the release of pigment into the dermis (Fig. 4.2). Copeman and Lewis (1973) described antibodies in the sera of patients with regressing halo naevi which cross reacted with melanoma cells but did not find antibodies of this kind in the sera of patients with other types of naevi. Miksche *et al.* (1975) found the lymphocytes of halo naevus patients capable of killing cultured melanoma cells. We have examined the leucocytes of three patients with halo naevi in the leucocyte migration assay and found them to be inhibited by extracts of their own tumours, extracts of allogeneic halo naevi and extracts of allogeneic malignant melanomas (Unpublished data).

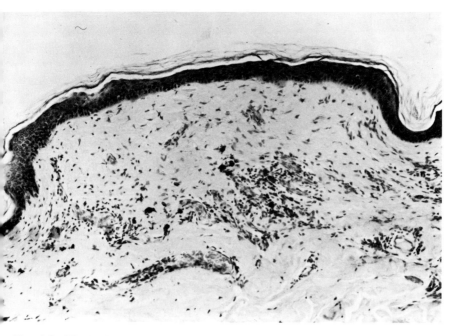

Fig. 4.2. Histological appearances of a regressed halo naevus. Haematoxylin and Eosin (× 125).

On the basis of this type of observation it has been claimed that "halo naevus" is a primary malignant melanoma undergoing regression, a suggestion which it is difficult to prove or refute. Certainly whatever the nature of the pre-existing melanocytic lesion it bears antigens with structural similarity to those of malignant melanoma.

BREAST DISEASE

In a comparable study of breast disease (Cochran *et al.*, 1974) we examined the leucocyte inhibitory activity of extracts of breast carcinoma, extracts of fibroadenomas and extracts of breasts showing mastopathic changes including some with prominent epitheliosis, a condition which is regarded as a hyperplasia of ductal epithelium (Table 4.1).

Breast cancer extracts selectively inhibited breast cancer patients' leucocytes but extracts of simple breast conditions inhibited leucocytes from the three groups of donors similarly infrequently. This suggests that the non-cancerous breast tissues examined carried no detectable antigens similar to those found on breast cancer cells. Also the leucocytes of patients with simple breast tumours or mastopathy were not sensitised to the tissues of these conditions, nor were they sensitised to breast cancer antigens. In a similar study McCoy *et al.* (1974) found an identical situation.

We have not examined women with breast carcinoma *in situ* (intraduct or intra-acinar carcinoma) but Black *et al.* (1976) reported that tumour directed cell mediated immunity was stronger in women with *in situ* breast cancer than in those with locally invasive or metastatic cancer.

In a limited study (Cochran *et al.*, 1974) we prepared tissue extracts from three areas of histologically normal breast adjacent to breast carcinomas. Two were inactive against breast cancer leucocytes and leucocytes from control individuals. The third preferentially inhibited the migration of breast cancer leucocytes (breast cancer leucocytes, 9/13 positive, control donors, 1/7 positive), suggesting that carcinogen exposed tissues, even those which remain morphologically unaltered, may express tumour associated antigens.

PROSTATIC DISEASE

Comparisons of normal prostatic tissue, prostates showing benign nodular hyperplasia and those with carcinoma have yielded interesting results. In an early study Flocks *et al.* (1960) found no antigenic differences between benign and malignant prostatic tissues. Ablin *et al.* (1970) subsequently reported three prostate related antigens; two tissue-specific antigens and one related to the enzyme acid phosphatase. In an extension of these studies it was reported that normal prostate markers are reduced or absent in benign nodular hyperplasia and prostatic carcinoma (Ablin, 1972).

Antigenic differences are certainly detectable in comparisons of benign, hyperplastic, premalignant and malignant tissues and further study of this rather underworked area seems likely to be rewarding.

Variations of Tumour Cell Antigens at Different Stages of Established Malignancy

One explanation of the decline in tumour directed immunity in patients with advancing malignancy is that originally immunogenic membrane structures are suppressed, altered or masked on the cells of metastatic tumours. Recent studies provide some support for this contention but it is not yet clear whether this phenomenon is the rule or only an exceptional occurrence.

IMMUNOLOGICAL STUDIES *IN VIVO* AND *IN VITRO*

Kjaer and Christensen (1977), using the leucocyte migration assay, reported extracts of metastatic renal carcinoma to be less antigenic than preparations of primary tumours from patients with no evidence of tumour spread. Leucocytes from patients whose tumours were weakly antigenic or non-antigenic were less likely to react against antigenic allogeneic tumours. Are such tumours of low antigenicity *ab initio*, which might aid evasion of host identification and facilitate spread or does low antigenicity of metastatic tumours result from the removal of strongly antigenic cells by selective pressures? Comparison of preparations from primary tumours and subsequent metastases should elucidate this. Black *et al.* (1976) provided indirect evidence of a stage related variation of tumour cell antigenicity by their observation that tumour-directed, cell-mediated immunity is more frequent in women with *in situ* breast carcinoma than in those with invasive or metastatic cancer. Roth *et al.* (1976) found that 3M KCl extracts of different melanoma metastases varied in their ability to induce delayed-type skin reactions and attributed this to antigenic disparities or variation in the content of skin reaction inhibitors.

We have examined the leucocyte migration inhibiting activity of 30 formalin-fixed single cell suspensions of melanomas from this standpoint. There was considerable variation in the specificity and activity of the preparations regardless of whether they were prepared from primary tumours, local recurrences, lymph node metastases or visceral metastases. Preparations from patients with advanced tumours were less active than those from patients with limited disease. We do not know whether this reduced activity is due to antigen loss or modification or to the presence of coating materials (Unpublished data).

MORPHOLOGICAL OBSERVATIONS

Morphological and histochemical studies indicate that tumours are not homogeneous in terms of cytology and function. In tumours preceded by a long *in situ* growth phase the development of invasive tumour may represent the evolution of cells with special characteristics. There is certainly an extreme behavioural difference between the cells of *in situ* malignancy and those of an invasive tumour which is often paralleled by cytological, ultra-structural and functional changes. Examples of this situation are the horizontal growth phase of lentigo maligna melanoma and superficial spreading melanoma, carcinoma *in situ* of the cervix uteri and skin and intraduct carcinoma of breast.

In situ malignancy is commonly associated with a dense infiltrate of "inflammatory" cells while invasive tumours often have a much reduced reactive component confined to the tumour periphery rather than infiltrating it. This is illustrated by lentigo maligna in which the cells, while pleomorphic are generally spindle shaped, usually show good melanogenesis and are often attended by an inflammatory reaction, while an associated vertically invasive malignant melanoma comprises cells which may be spindle shaped or epithelioid or both, may or may not show melanogenesis and may attract relatively few inflammatory cells (Fig. 2.8). The importance of variations in lymphocellular infiltrates depends on the validity of current interpretations of their nature, role and significance. In the absence of extraneous antigenic stimulation by infection or the introduction of BCG, vaccinia virus or DNCB as local immunotherapy, the infiltrating cells may represent an immune response to tumour-associated antigens. It is difficult to interpret the cytological composition of the infiltrates as other than that of an immuno-logical reaction. The evidence for their constituting an aggressive anti-tumour response is weaker than one would wish, but there is evidence of transfer of information from the tumour cells to closely applied lympho-reticular cells as would occur in the afferent limb of an immune response. It seems reasonable that this may be due in part to neoantigens on the tumour cells. If so, the decline in cellular reaction around invasive tumours may be due to the selective evolution of tumour cells in which antigenic disparity is insufficient to induce or maintain an immune response. Laboratory studies of this have been inconclusive as the cells of peritumoral infiltrates have proved difficult to investigate with current techniques. Other interpretations of this situation are discussed in Chapter 5.

Further evidence of selective variation of tumour cells is provided by invasive tumours in which two or more separate populations of cells exist

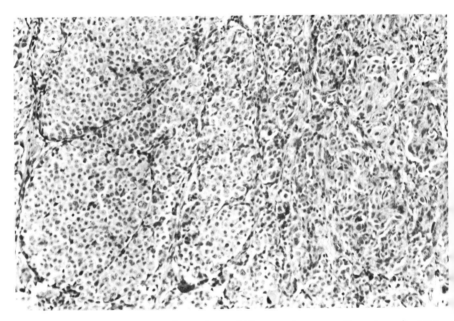

Fig. 4.3. Intralesional transformation within a primary malignant melanoma. Haematoxylin and Eosin (× 200).

with strikingly different morphology, functional capacity and ultrastructural morphology (intralesional transformation) and which have associated "inflammatory" infiltrates of strikingly different magnitude (Fig. 4.3). Again, while separate tumour metastases may be comprised of cell populations which are identical in morphology and function, they may differ widely in appearance, function and lymphoreticular response suggesting that selective evolution has occurred.

The subject of tumour cell evolution in relation to varying clinical stage is discussed in depth, using malignant melanoma as a model, by Clark *et al.* (1975).

References

Abelev, G. I. (1963). *Acta UICC* **19**, 80.
Abelev, G. I. (1971). *Adv. Cancer Res.* **14**, 295.
Ablin, R. J., Bronson, P., Soanes, W. A. and Witebsky, E. (1970). *J. Immunol.* **104**, 1329.
Ablin, R. J. (1972). *Cancer* **29**, 1570-1574.
Alpert, E., Pinn, V. W. and Isselbacher, K. J. (1971). *New Engl. J. Med.* **285**, 1058.
Andersen, V., Bjerrum, O., Bendixen, G., Schiødt, T. and Dissing, I. (1970). *Int. J. Cancer* **5**, 357-363.
Aurelian, L., Strandberg, J. D., Melendez, L. V. and Johnson, L. A. (1971). *Science* **174**, 704-707.
Aurelian, L. (1974). *Cancer Res.* **34**, 1126-1135.
Aurelian, L. and Strnad, B. C. (1976). *Cancer Res.* **36**, 810-820.
Baldwin, R. W. and Barker, C. R. (1967). *Int. J. Cancer* **2**, 355.
Baldwin, R. W., Price, M. R. and Robins, R. A. (1973). *Brit. J. Cancer* **28**, Suppl. 1, 37-47.
Bell, C. E. and Seetharam, S. (1976). *Int. J. Cancer* **18**, 605-611.
Benacerraf, B. and McDevitt, H. O. (1972). *Science* **175**, 273.
Black, M. M., Leis, H. P., Shore, B. and Zachrau, R. E. (1974a). *Cancer* **33**, 952-958.
Black, M. M., Moore, D. H., Shore, B., Zachrau, R. E. and Leis, H. P. (1974b). *Cancer Res.* **34**, 1054-1060.
Black, M. M., Zachrau, R. E., Shore, B. and Leis, H. P. (1976). *Cancer Res.* **36**, 769-774.
Brawn, R. J. (1970). *Int. J. Cancer* **6**, 245.
Brown, F. C. and Tan, E. M. (1973). *Cancer Res.* **33**, 2030-2033.
Burkitt, D. (1963). *Int. Rev. exptl. Pathol.* **2**, 67-138.
Burrows, D. (1958). *Brit. med. J.* **1**, 368-370.
Castro, J. E. (1972). *Nature (New Biol.)* **239**, 83.
Char, D. H., Hollinshead, A. C., Cogan, D. G., Ballintine, E. J., Hogan, M. J. and Herberman, R. B. (1974). *New Engl. J. Med.* **291**, 274-277.
Clark, D. A., Necheles, T. F., Nathanson, L., Whitten, D., Silverman, E. and Flowers, A. (1974). *In* "Immunological parameters of host-tumour relationships", Volume III (D. W. Weiss, Ed.). Academic Press, New York and London.
Clark, W. H., Ainsworth, A. M., Bernardino, E. A., Yang, C.-H., Mihm, M. C. and Reed, R. J. (1975). *Seminars in Oncology* **2**, 83-103.

Cochran, A. J., Spilg, W. G. S., Mackie, R. M. and Thomas, C. E. (1972). *Brit. med. J.* **4,** 67-70.

Cochran, A. J., Grant, R. M., Spilg, W. G. S., Mackie, R. M., Ross, C. E., Hoyle, D. E. and Russell, J. M. (1974). *Int. J. Cancer* **14,** 19-25.

Coggin, J. H. and Anderson, N. G. (1974). *Adv. Cancer Res.* **19,** 105-165.

Cohen, D., Gurner, B. W. and Coombs, R. R. A. (1971). *Brit. J. exp. Pathol.* **52,** 447-451.

Cohen, I. R., Wekerle, H. and Feldman, M. (1974). *In* "Immunological Parameters of host-tumour relationships" (D. Weiss, Ed.) 210-218. Academic Press, New York and London.

Copeman, P. W. M., Lewis, M. G., Phillips, T. M. and Elliott, P. G. (1973). *Brit. J. Derm.* **88,** 127-137.

Criss, W. E. (1971). *Cancer Res.* **31,** 1523.

Currie, G. A. and Basham, C. (1972). *Brit. J. Cancer* **26,** 427-438.

Currie, G. A. and Alexander, P. (1974). *Brit. J. Cancer* **29,** 72-75.

deSchryver, A., Friberg, S., Klein, G., Henle, W., Henle, G., deThe, G., Clifford, P. and Ho, H. C. (1969). *Clin. Exper. Immunol.* **5,** 443-459.

Detre, S. I. and Gazet, J. C. (1973). *Brit. J. Cancer* **28,** 412.

Dmochowski, L. and Bowen, J. M. (1973). Proc. 7th National Cancer Conference, Los Angeles, pp 697-710.

Edynak, E. M., Hirshaut, Y. and Bernard, M. (1972). *J. nat. Cancer Inst.,* **48,** 1137.

Epstein, M. A., Achong, B. G. and Barr, Y. M. (1964). *Lancet* **1,** 702-703.

Epstein, M. A., Hunt, R. D. and Rabin, H. (1973). *Int. J. Cancer* **12,** 309-318.

Everleigh, J. W. (1972). *In* "Embryonic foetal antigens in Cancer" (N. G. Anderson and J. H. Coggin, Jr. Eds.) Vol. 2, 133. U.S. Dept. Commerce, Springfield, Virginia.

Federman, J. L., Lewis, M. G. and Clark, W. H. (1974). *J. nat. Cancer Inst.* **52,** 587.

Fishman, W. H., Inglis, N. I., Stolbach, L. L. and Krant, M. (1968). *Cancer Res.* **28,** 150.

Flocks, R. H., Urich, V. C., Patel, C. A. and Opitz, J. M. (1960). *J. Urol.* **84,** 134.

Franks, C. R., Perkins, F. T. and Holmes, J. T. (1973). *Nature* **243,** 91.

Frenkel, N., Roizman, B., Cassai, E. and Nahmias, A. J. (1972). *Proc. nat. Acad. Sci. U.S.* **69,** 3784-3789.

Giovanella, B. C., Yim, S. O., Stehlin, J. S. and Williams, L. J. (1972). *J. nat. Cancer Inst.* **48,** 1531-1533.

Globerson, A. and Feldman, M. (1964). *J. nat. Cancer Inst.* **32,** 1229.

Gold, P. and Freedman, S. O. (1965). *J. exp. Med.* **122,** 467.

Goudie, R. B. and McCallum, H. M. (1963). *Lancet* **2,** 1035-1038.

Grace, J. T. and Lehoczky, A. (1959). *Surgery* **46,** 238-246.

Green, H. (1950). *Yale J. Biol. Med.* **22,** 611-620.

Greenblatt, M. and Shubik, P. (1968). *J. nat. Cancer Inst.* **41,** 111.

Habel, K. (1961). *Proc. Soc. exp. Biol. Med.* **106,** 722.

Hackett, E. and Gardonyi, E. (1960). *Brit. med. J.* **1,** 1785-1787.

Halterman, R. (1973). *New Engl. J. Med.* **187,** 1272-1274.

Harris, R., Viza, D., Todd, R., Phillips, J., Sugar, R., Jennison, R. F., Marriott, G. and Gleeson, M. H. (1971). *Nature* **233,** 556.

Hellström, K. E. (1969). *Int. J. Cancer* **4,** 601.

Henle, G. and Henle, W. (1966). *Trans. N.Y. Acad. Sci.* **29,** 71-79.

Henle, W., Diehl, V., Kohn, G., Zur Hausen, H. and Henle, G. (1967). *Science* **157,** 1064-1065.

Henle, G., Henle, W. and Diehl, V. (1968). *Proc. nat. Acad. Sci. U.S.* **59,** 94-101.

Henle, G., Henle, W., Clifford, P., Diehl, V., Kafuko, G. W., Kirya, B. G., Klein, G., Morrow, R. H., Munube, G. M. R., Pike, P., Tukei, P. M. and Ziegler, J. L. (1969). *J. nat. Cancer Inst.* **43**, 1147-1158.

Hersey, P., Morgan, G., Stone, D. E., McCarthy, W. H. and Milton, G. W. (1977a). *Lancet* **1**, 451-452.

Hersey, P., Honeyman, M., Edwards, A., Adams, E. and McCarthy, W. H. (1977b) *Int. J. Cancer* **18**, 564.

Hirszfeld, L., Halber, W. and Laskowski, J. (1929). *Ztschr. Immunitäts.* **64**, 61-80.

Hollinshead, A. C. and Herberman, R. B. (1973). *In* "Proceedings of the Second International Symposium on Cancer Detection and Prevention" (G. Maltoni, Ed.) 102-104. Elsevier, New York.

Hollinshead, A. C., Jaffurs, W. T., Alpert, L. K., Harris, J. E. and Herberman, R. B. (1974a). *Cancer Res.* **34**, 2961-2968.

Hollinshead, A. C., Herberman, R. B., Jaffurs, W. J., Alpert, L. K., Minten, J. P. and Harris, J. E. (1974b). *Cancer* **34**, 1235-1243.

Hollinshead, A. C., Stewart, T. H. M. and Herberman, R. B. (1974c). *J. nat. Cancer Inst.* **52**, 327-338.

Hollinshead, A. C. and Stewart, T. H. M. *In* "Proceedings of the Third International Symposium on Cancer Detection and Prevention". (In Press.)

Ivaskova, E., Jakoubkova, J., Zavadil, M., Schneid, V., Koldovsky, P. and Ivanyi, P. (1969). *Transplant Proc.* **1**, 80.

Johansson, B., Klein, G., Henle, W. and Henle, G. (1970). *Int. J. Cancer* **6**, 450-462.

Johansson, B., Klein, G., Henle, W. and Henle, G. (1971). *Int. J. Cancer* **8**, 475-486.

Kjaer, M. and Christensen, N. (1976). *Cancer Immunol. Immunother.* **2**, 41.

Klein, G., Sjögren, H. O., Klein, E. and Hellström, K. E. (1960). *Cancer Res.* **22**, 955.

Kufe, D., Hehlmann, R. and Spiegelman, S. (1973). *Proc. nat. Acad. Sci. U.S.* **70**, 5-9.

Lappé, M. A. (1968). *J. nat. Cancer Inst.* **40**, 823-846.

Lehner, T. (1970). *Brit. J. Cancer* **24**, 442.

Levine, P. H., Ablashi, D. V., Bernard, C. W., Carbone, P. P. and Waggoner, D. E. (1970). *Proc. Amer. Assoc. Cancer Res.* **11**, 49.

Levine, P. H. (1972a). *Cancer* **30**, 875.

Levine, P. H., Merrill, D. A., Bethlenfalvay, N. C., Dabich, L., Stevens, D. A. and Waggoner, D. E. (1972b). *Blood* **38**, 479-481.

Makari, I. (1958). *Brit. med. J.* **2**, 358-361.

Mann, J. (1972). *Science* **174**, 1136-1137.

Manuelidis, E. E. (1971). *Yale J. Biol. Med.* **43**, 307-322.

Metzgar, R. S. (1972). *Science* **178**, 986.

Metzgar, R. S., Bergoc, P. M., Moreno, M. A. and Siegler, H. F. (1973). *J. nat. Cancer Inst.* **50**, 1065-1068.

Miksche, M., Cerni, C., Kokoschka, E. and Gebhart, W. (1976). *Pigment Cell* **2**, 264-272.

Milgrom, F., Humphrey, L. J., Tønder, O., Yasuda, J. and Witebsky, E. (1968). *Int. Arch. Allergy* **33**, 478-492.

Miller, D. R. (1969). *Int. J. Haematol.* **17**, 103.

Morgensen, B., Kissmeyer-Nielsen, F. and Hauge, M. (1969). *Transplant. Proc.* **1**, 76.

Morrow, R. H., Gutesohn, N. and Smith, P. G. (1976). *Cancer Res.* **36**, 667-669.

McCoy, J. L., Jerome, L. F., Dean, J. H., Cannon, G. B., Alford, T. D., Doering, T. and Herberman, R. B. (1974). *J. nat. Cancer Inst.* **53**, 11-17.

Niederman, J. C., McCollum, R. W., Henle, G. and Henle, W. (1968). *J. Amer. med. Ass.* **203,** 205-209.

Old, L. J., Boyse, E. A., Clark, D. A. and Carswell, E. A. (1962). *Ann. N. Y. Acad. Sci.* **101,** 80.

Palmer, A. E., London, W. T., Nahmias, A. J., Naib, Z. M., Tunca, J., Fuccillo, D. A., Ellenberg, J. H. and Sever, J. L. (1976). *Cancer Res.* **36,** 807-809.

Parmiani, G. and Della Porta, G. (1973). *Nature (New Biol.)* **241,** 26.

Pope, J. H., Horne, M. K. and Scott, W. (1968). *Int. J. Cancer* **3,** 857-866.

Povlsen, C. O. and Rygaard, J. (1971). *Acta Path. et Microbiol Scand. A.* **79,** 159.

Prehn, R. T. and Main, J. M. (1957). *J. nat. Cancer Inst.* **18,** 768.

Prehn, R. T. and Slemmer, G. L. (1967). *In* "Endogenous factors influencing Host-Tumour Balance" (R. W. Wissler, T. L. Dao and S. W. Woods, Eds.) 185-190. University of Chicago Press.

Priori, E. S., Seman, G., Dmochowski, L., Gallagher, H. S. and Anderson, D. E. (1971). *Cancer* **28,** 1462-1471.

Rapin, A. M. C. and Burger, M. M. (1974). *Adv. Cancer Res.* **10,** 1-92.

Reynoso, G., Chu, T. M. and Holyoke, D. (1972). *J. Amer. med. Ass.* **220,** 361.

Richmond, R. E. and Morton, D. L. (1974). *J. Reticuloendothel. Soc.* **16,** 8.

Roth, J. A., Slocum, H. K., Pellegrino, M. A., Holmes, E. C. and Reisfeld, R. A. (1976). *Cancer Res.* **36,** 2360-2364.

Ruoslahti, E., Seppälä, M., Vuopio, P., Saksela, E. and Peltokallio, P. (1972). *J. nat. Cancer Inst.* **49,** 623-630.

Salinas, F. A., Smith, J. A. and Hanna, M. G. (1972). *In* "Embryonic and fetal antigens in Cancer" (N. G. Anderson and J. H. Coggin, Jr. Eds.) Vol. 2, 187. U.S. Dept. Commerce, Springfield, Virginia.

Schlom, J. and Spiegelman, S. (1973). *Amer. J. Clin. Path.* **60,** 44-56.

Segall, A., Weiler, O., Genin, J., Lacour, J. and Lacour, F. (1972). *Int. J. Cancer* **9,** 417-425.

Singer, K., Chernott, A. I. and Singer, L. (1951). *Blood* **6,** 413.

Smith, J. B. and O'Neill, R. T. (1971). *Amer. J. med.* **51,** 767-771.

Takahashi, M. and Yamanishi, K. (1974). *Virology,* **61,** 306-311.

Tal, C., Dishon, T. and Gross, J. (1964). *Brit. J. Cancer* **18,** 111.

Tatarinov, Y. (1964). *Vopr. Med. Khim.* **10,** 90.

Thomson, D. M. P., Krupey, J., Freedman, S. O. and Gold, P. (1969). *Proc. nat. Acad. Sci. U.S.* **64,** 161.

Thunold, S., Abeyounis, C. J., Milgrom, F. and Witebsky, E. (1970). *Int. Arch. Allergy* **38,** 260-268.

Tønder, O., Humphrey, L. J. and Morso, P. (1975). *Cancer* **35,** 580-587.

Tønder, O. and Thunold, S. (1973). *Scand. J. Immunol.* **2,** 207-215.

Turk, J. L. (1969). *In* "Immunology in Clinical Medicine". Heinemann, London.

Vaidya, A. B., Black, M. M., Dion, A. S. and Moore, D. H. (1974). *Nature* **249,** 565-567.

Weintraub, B. D. and Rosen, S. W. (1971). *J. Clin. Endocrinol.* **32,** 94.

Wilson, N. I. L., Ross, C. E., Mackie, R. M. and Cochran, A. J. (Submitted to *Cancer Immunol. Immunother.*)

Witebsky, E. (1930). *Klin. Wchnschr.* **9,** 58-63.

Zilber, L. A. and Abelev, G. I. (1968). "The Virology and Immunology of Cancer" 211-220. Pergamon Press, London.

5

The Paradox of Tumour Growth in the Presence of Tumour-Directed Immunity

In the face of tumour-directed immune reactions, demonstrable by autograft rejection and delayed cutaneous hypersensitivity *in vivo* and by a range of assays for humoral and cellular immunity *in vitro* it is perplexing that cancer is so often an aggressive and lethal disease. Many more or less plausible explanations have been advanced for this apparent paradox, but despite the key importance of an understanding of the mechanisms involved, they remain incompletely understood.

We do not know the extent to which (if at all) tumour associated antigens on human tumours function as rejection inducing antigens in the manner of transplantation antigens in allografts. TAA may merely be interesting epiphenomena and the immune responses which they evoke may have no significant capacity to cause cytostatic or cytotoxic effects. If so these responses are merely a curious irrelevance and tumour progression in the face of such responses is no longer paradoxical. In animals it is relatively simple to assay transplantable tumours for immunogenicity and induced immune responses for anti-tumour activity in immunoprotection experiments. In man, the fact that tumour autografts must be of considerable size to achieve progressive growth (Brunschwig *et al.*, 1965) points to the existence of concomitant immunity (Gershon *et al.*, 1967) and some tumour rejection potential.

It is of course possible that the body is outstandingly efficient at protecting itself against cancer. If the advocates of immune surveillance are correct we all continually develop mutant cells including some with malignant potential which are recognised and destroyed by the reticuloendothelial cells. The development of clinically detectable cancer in this context represents a single failure against which may be set numerous previous successes where emergent malignant clones have been identified and destroyed. Carcinoma *in situ* may be present for many years (up to 30 years in the case of *lentigo maligna*) before an invasive tumour develops, although the cytology of the preinvasive lesion from its earliest stages would warrant a diagnosis of overt malignancy if the cells had escaped from their normal anatomical compartment. These lesions are usually associated with an "inflammatory" infiltrate which may be an index of powerful host mechanisms which, by restraining the cancer cells from invasion, will extend the tumour bearer's life. The difference between *in situ* and invasive cancer might equally result from the acquisition or expression by the tumour cells of new special characteristics which permit invasion.

The balance between tumour aggressiveness and host defences is likely to be a fine one and dominance of one or other side of this equilibrium will vary from time to time. Excessive imbalance may determine progression or halting of tumour growth and spread. The reappearance of cancer after prolonged latency is probably an example of the effects of major imbalance of this kind. The factors which trigger this event are unknown but may include immunological depression, either endogenous or a deliberate or inadvertent sequel of therapy, a situation similar to the redevelopment of tuberculosis from latent mycobacteria in patients on steroid therapy.

There are two major situations to be considered in which tumour growth may be free of immunologically based host-control. Firstly a tumour may not naturally induce an immune response at any time and secondly a tumour-evoked immune response which is initially of significant strength and anti-tumour activity may subsequently weaken or be totally lost. Although the end result of these two situations is the same it is important to distinguish between them since approaches to rectifying them seem likely to be quite separate, involving induction of immunity and perhaps of selective immune capacity in the former case and the restitution and amplification of a preexisting capability in the other.

Tumours not Associated with a Tumour-Directed Immune Reaction

While it is simplest to conceive of tumour-directed immunity in terms of an all or none situation it may be that a weak response has as little anti-tumour activity as no response or that weak reactions may even enhance tumour growth (Prehn, 1976).

GENETIC FACTORS

The characteristics of the immune response to any given antigen, including tumour antigens (Lilly and Pincus, 1973; Muhlbock and Dux, 1974) are modified by "Ir" (immune responsiveness) genes active at all stages of the immune response. By dictating a weak or negative response these genes are one cause of specific genetic unresponsiveness. Absence of the genetic apparatus necessary for a response to certain antigens has also been suggested (Laroye, 1973). Since TAA are T lymphocyte dependent, genetically determined absence or functional abnormality of T lymphocytes would also be associated with a nil response. Non responsiveness could also result from maturation linked tolerance, especially to embryonal tumours.

ANATOMICAL FACTORS

Tumours arising in sites from which antigen cannot readily escape or the cells of the afferent limb of the immune response penetrate (privileged sites) would induce either a suboptimal or no response.

TUMOUR CELL CHARACTERISTICS

Tumour cells totally devoid of neoantigens or on which TAA are totally and continually masked would be non-immunogenic. The immunogenic strength of TAA varies with the nature of the inducing carcinogen, its dose and route of administration and the latent period between carcinogen exposure and tumour development. The development or failure of an immune response to TAA will thus always depend on the subtle interplay of these factors.

For the very practical purpose of obtaining positive reactions much experimental work in animal tumour immunology has concerned strongly antigenic tumours to the relative neglect of non-antigenic or weakly antigenic systems. This, though understandable, is probably counterproductive from the standpoint of human tumour immunology, as many human tumours seem relatively weakly autoimmunogenic. Studies of more relevant animal models are therefore now attracting more interest (Klein and Klein, 1977).

Tumours Associated with an Immune Response which Fails Secondarily or is Circumvented

The factors involved in tumour escape from host control, are conveniently considered as those relating to the tumour bearing host, those relating to the tumour cells and aspects of the manner in which host and tumour cells react with each other.

FACTORS RELATING TO THE TUMOUR BEARING HOST

Immunological integrity

Immunological integrity, the possession of all components of the immunological apparatus functioning normally, is associated with a relatively low incidence of cancer. The efficiency of the immune system can, however, be affected by a remarkably wide range of influences ranging from physiological variations in endocrine activity to highly immune-depressant medicaments. The extent of the effects observed varies from mild and transient alterations in lymphocyte performance *in vitro*, without overt effects on host resistance *in vivo*, to massive prolonged depression of the ability to combat even organisms of low pathogenicity. It is therefore likely that each individual suffers numerous periods of variable susceptibility to the development of cancer (and other diseases).

After middle life malignant disease becomes increasingly frequent with advancing *age*. This may merely be the result of the accumulation of exposure to different carcinogens but it is also possible that, with increasing age there is a decline in the efficiency of the immune system which may permit the emergence and development of malignant clones. There is certainly an age related decline in the lymphocytic response to mitogens such as PHA, in skin test reactivity to recall antigens, and perhaps also in the primary response to synthetic antigens such as dinitrochlorobenzene. *Endocrine factors* influence immune functions directly via the interaction of steroid and other hormones with lymphoid cells and indirectly through the metabolic effects of endocrine diseases such as diabetes mellitus and thyrotoxicosis. Lung cancers which produce "inappropriate" ACTH have a worse prognosis than non-secretory tumours in that they spread early and widely, possibly due to immune suppression by excess adrenocortical hormones from the tumour product stimulated adrenal cortex. The transient decline of lymphocyte responsiveness *in vitro* during the immediate postoperative period (Cochran *et al.*, 1973) seems likely to be a result of the endocrine sequelae of surgery. *Diseases other than cancer* may induce immune depression, either by a direct effect on the cells of the reticulo-endothelial system (e.g. severe infections) or via the production and accumulation of toxic substances (e.g. uraemia) or by necessitating the use of *therapeutic agents* which inhibit immune functions (e.g. steroids or cytotoxic agents). *Tumours* themselves may cause immune suppression as may chemical carcinogens (Malmgren *et al.*., 1952; Stjernswärd, 1969) and oncogenic viruses (Peterson *et al.*, 1963; Cremer *et al.*, 1966). The situation with oncogenic viruses is especially interesting. Feline leukaemia virus, for instance, is capable of this activity and whether or not an exposed cat develops leukaemia, is to some extent dependent upon the degree of immune suppression induced by the virus (Essex *et al.*, 1971). *Physical factors* such as ionising radiations may also strongly influence the immune system.

Tolerance

The newborn child may possibly be uniquely susceptible to carcinogenesis in that even strongly antigenic agents if transmitted vertically from the mother *in utero* or encountered in the early postnatal period may be considered as self and treated as tolerogenic rather than immunogenic. Such agents may retain their carcinogenic effect and tumours result, the age of their emergence depending upon the dose of carcinogen and its latent period (Klein and Klein, 1964). It has been claimed, for instance, that children born to women pregnant during influenza epidemics have an increased risk of developing leukaemia (Stewart *et al.*, 1958; Hakulinen *et al.*, 1973). Low zone tolerance may be important in the "sneaking through" hypothesis discussed below and high zone tolerance may be induced where tumour volume is large and the rate of tumour antigen release is high.

Absolute or relative deficiencies of immunocompetent effector cells

A reduction in the net effectiveness of the immune system could arise from an absolute deficiency in immunocompetent cells or from a reduction of the functional efficiency of a normal number of immunocytes and, if associated with carcinogen exposure might facilitate tumour development. The former situation could be exemplified by immunological deficiency syndromes with a (selective) lymphocyte deficit or possibly by the lymphopenia which follows radiotherapy, although in this latter situation an element of functional derangement seems likely also to be involved.

If antigen specific T-cell mediated cytotoxicity is a main force in tumour control its role seems likely to be transient as the amplification of specifically sensitised T cells will be limited by suppressor cells and the immune suppressive effects of growing tumours. A progressively growing tumour with a steady antigenic profile seems likely to outstrip the cytotoxic capacity of the amplified T-cell population relatively easily, producing a situation of relative effector cell deficiency. K cell killing of antibody coated tumour cells then becomes of paramount importance, although this mechanism too may be evanescent, as a relative deficiency of antitumour antibody also seems possible. If situations of relative deficiency were readily identifiable passive replacement with lymphoid cells or antibodies might provide a rational approach to their management.

Even with a full complement of immunologically competent cells the conjunction of carcinogen exposure with a second disease process may alter the manner in which an immunogenic carcinogen is handled (immunological preoccupation). The resultant abnormal host-carcinogen interaction may result in malignant transformation of susceptible cells, survival of the transformed cells and their progression to a tumour. This concept seems particularly applicable to oncogenic viruses and may explain in part sporadic oncogenesis by viruses which do not cause tumours in the overwhelming majority of virus-exposed individuals belonging to the natural host species.

FACTORS RELATING TO THE TUMOUR

As a tumour develops selection pressures dictate the survival of those cells best adapted to the host. This may be by the outgrowth of the single clone of cells which possesses the most resistant phenotype or of several clones with phenotypes which differ from each other in some respects but are all compatible with survival. Studies of tumour cell characteristics such as surface Ig, iso-enzymes and chromosomal markers suggest that the majority of tumours are monoclonal (Friedman and Fialkow, 1976). However without extensive comparison of multiple markers at different stages in tumour progression the true extent of antigenic diversity within primary tumours and between them and their *in situ* phase and their metastases cannot be accurately assessed. The characteristics which favour survival, invasion and metastasis largely remain a mystery, but attempts are in progress to investigate some which, on the basis of current thinking, seem relevant.

Tumour cell antigenicity

Tumour cells devoid of detectable TAA or with weakly immunogenic TAA are clearly at an advantage *if the immune response to TAA is cytostatic or cytotoxic*. The same is true of tumour cells bearing strongly immunogenic TAA if these are substantially covered by a masking coat or blocking factors (see below). However, even a tumour cell bearing strongly immunogenic exposed TAA will be at risk only if the tumour host possesses the genetic apparatus for recognising the TAA as foreign and for mounting a significant immune reaction to them. This crucial point has been elegantly demonstrated in a mouse model by Kiessling *et al.* (1975).

The capacity to modify antigenicity

The capacity to modify an obtrusive antigenic profile may make the difference between the survival of a tumour and its extinction. Antigen expression at the cell membrane may be altered by immune attack *in vivo* (e.g. growth in a presensitised host) or *in vitro* (e.g. cultured cells growing in medium supplemented with antibodies of appropriate specificity) (Fenyö *et al.*, 1968). This may be due to cessation of transcription of the appropriate gene leading to *antigenic deletion* at the membrane or to modification of the rate of synthesis of the appropriate antigen leading to *antigenic modulation*. The expression of membrane antigens varies throughout the cell-cycle (Cikes, 1970). Variations in cell-cycle kinetics of a tumour cell population may thus produce a significant change in tumour immunogenicity based on quantitative rather than qualitative changes in TAA expression. Selection of tumour cells for a bland antigenic profile in the face of strong anti-tumour immunity is clearly another possibility. The monoclonality of many tumours may be interpreted as against this, but without serial studies of the antigens under attack *immune selection* cannot at present be excluded.

An alternative to antigenic modification or deletion is the production by the tumour cells of coating materials such as sialomucins which will overlay and effectively hide TAA from recognition and the effects of specifically sensitised effector cells. A similar result might follow the coating of tumour cells with non-cytotoxic antibodies, though these, if of the appropriate IgG subclass, might be expected to prime the cells to K cell attack. This problem would be overcome if, as Keisari and Witz have suggested (Chapter 3), the attached antibody molecules are cleaved by proteolytic enzymes, removing the Fc portions and leaving the Fab portions attached to and occluding the determinant sites. Prior to causing the death of antibody coated target cells K cells must attach to them by Fc receptors, thus cells bearing only Fab fragments would be immune from this form of immune attack. The kinetics of molecular synthesis and distribution in tumour cell membranes must obviously have a bearing on tumour cell survival and on the impact of immune attack on them. Relatively few studies of this kind have as yet been undertaken in human tumours but there is current interest in the extent and rate of capping (movement of antigen-bound antibody to the cell pole prior to endocytosis) of antibody bound to membrane located antigens (Yefenof and Klein, 1974) and in the shedding of membrane antigens, including TAA, into the extracellular fluids, either as part of physiological membrane turnover or following interaction with antibody (Currie and Basham, 1972). Other features such as antigen frequency, distribution and depth in the membrane are also likely to be of interest.

Immunoresistance

This interesting concept derives from the observation that cells vary in their sensitivity to lymphocyte mediated cytotoxicity *in vitro* (Hellström, 1959; Klein and Möller, 1963). It seems likely, although difficult to prove, that cells exhibit a similarly variable susceptibility to immune attack *in vivo*. The effect is partly due to surface antigen concentration, and this is true for transplantation antigens and TAA (Fenyö *et al.*, 1968; Tevethia *et al.*, 1971). However other factors are involved since immunoresistance and antigen concentrations are not always directly associated (Friberg *et al.*, 1973). Studies with virus-fused hybrid cell tumours further support the existence of several mechanisms of immunoresistance since the characteristic behaves as a dominant trait in some hybrids and in a recessive manner in others (Fenyö *et al.*, 1971; Klein *et al.*, 1970). Immunoresistance may well be a major factor in tumour cell survival in the presence of antitumour immunity and clearly merits the more detailed study it is now receiving.

The physical distribution of tumour cells

Tumour cells organised in well vascularised masses seem less susceptible to immune attack than those in small clumps or dispersed singly in the tissues or body fluids. Apart from any consideration of the volume and number of cells present in tumours it is obviously more difficult for antibodies and effector cells to achieve significant penetration of tightly arranged tumour cell masses. It may be that anti-tumour (concomitant) immunity has as one of its main roles the destruction of separated tumour cells and in this manner limits the establishment of metastases. This role might serve to explain the often repeated observations of relatively large numbers of circulating tumour cells early in malignancy, without a commensurately large establishment of metastatic deposits (Chapter 2).

FACTORS RELATING TO THE INTERACTION OF TUMOUR CELLS AND HOST

Tumour growth rate

A tumour which grows very rapidly may outstrip the capacity of the immune system to respond to it and lead to immune paralysis or high zone tolerance. In animal studies very small and very large inocula of antigenic tumour cells may grow progressively where intermediate numbers fail. This phenomenon which is rather quaintly called "sneaking through" (Old *et al.*, 1962) appears to depend on the balance between tumour growth rate and the speed with which a significant response may be mounted against it. Since "sneaking through" must occur very early in the development of a tumour it would seem nearly impossible to investigate it in man.

Tumour enhancement and blocking

In animal experiments various immunological manipulations have been associated with and probably cause increased tumour growth and spread (*immunological enhancement*). It is a near constant feature of studies of active specific and active non specific immune therapy in animals that while some combinations of agent, route of administration and timing may reduce tumour takes or progression others, often very little different from the "effective" regimen, have the opposite effect. It is clearly very worrying, that immunological manipulations, including those designed to reduce tumour progression may instead have a contrary effect and much effort has been expended to identify the factors involved. The natural variability of human malignant disease makes it difficult to identify enhancement in the individual patient other than in a randomised clinical trial.

In animals it is possible to enhance tumour growth by treating tumour bearing animals with noncytotoxic anti-tumour antibody, which appears to impede the effector cells of the tumour directed immune response (for review see Baldwin *et al.*, 1973). This activity has accordingly been termed "blocking" and is analogous to the inhibitory activities of anti-H-2 antibodies described by Möller and Möller (1962).

There have been numerous investigations of cancer patients' sera for evidence of blocking activity and attempts to identify the active materials in positive sera. Most studies have examined sera for their capacity to abrogate lymphocyte mediated killing or inhibition of tumour target cells *in vitro* (see Hellström and Hellström, 1974 for review). By analogy with animal studies it was initially held that the active material was noncytotoxic anti-tumour antibody, which, by combining with membrane located antigens, prevented sensitised lymphocytes or *cytotoxic* antibodies from attaching to them and inducing cytolysis (Figure 5.1A). Unfortunately this simple hypothesis is probably only correct in few specialised situations (see below). Numerous studies have shown that blocking activity is high when actively growing tumour is present, at which time anti-tumour antibodies are present at only moderate concentration. Blocking becomes undetectable shortly after tumour excision at a time when the titre of anti-tumour antibodies increases. In fact post-excision or post-regression sera possess "unblocking" activities, and if mixed with blocking sera neutralise the blocking effect (Hellström *et al.*, 1973).

For a patient's sera to have blocking activity the presence of tumour tissue is necessary. Subsequent studies have suggested that the component donated by the tumour cell is TAA, released spontaneously or complexed with anti-tumour antibody after combination at the cell membrane. Sjögren *et al.* (1971) subjected blocking sera to low pH (a standard technique for dissociating antigen-antibody complexes) and subsequent millipore filtration. After restoration to neutral pH neither the high molecular weight components retained above the filter nor low molecular weight material passed through the filter were capable of blocking. Recombination of the two fractions restored blocking activity, suggesting strongly that, in this situation, blocking was due to immune complexes. Using a similar approach of acid separation and filtration Mukojima *et al.* (1973) showed it to increase the titre of antibodies in pre-recurrence sera from Burkitt lymphoma patients.

Immune complexes seem most likely to act either by free antigenic determinants attaching to specific antigen receptors on lymphocytes (Fig. 5.1B) or by attachment of Fc portions of antibody molecules in the complexes to Fc receptors on lymphocytes or tumour cells (Fig. 5.1C). This mechanism would also interfere with non sensitised effector cells including K cells and macrophages, the only requirement being the presence of an Fc receptor. Immune complexes in antigen excess would also combine with specific antibodies, including cytotoxic antibodies and those capable of priming

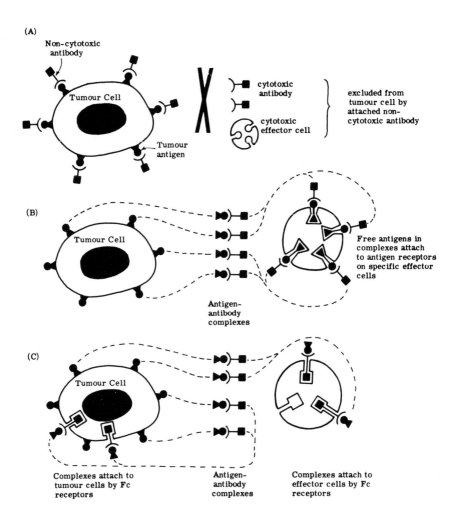

Fig. 5.1. Diagram of postulated mechanisms whereby tumour directed antibodies and specifically sensitised lymphocytes may be excluded from contact with tumour cells.

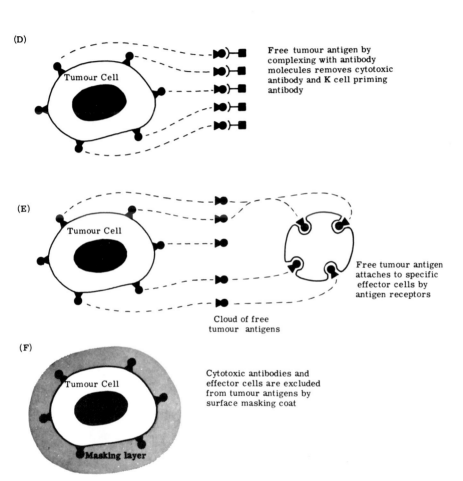

(D) Free tumour antigen by complexing with antibody molecules removes cytotoxic antibody and K cell priming antibody

(E) Free tumour antigen attaches to specific effector cells by antigen receptors

Cloud of free tumour antigens

(F) Cytotoxic antibodies and effector cells are excluded from tumour antigens by surface masking coat

Fig. 5.1 (cont.)

tumour cells to K cell attack (Fig. 5.1D). According to this scheme unblocking sera would neutralise blocking complexes in which there was antigen excess by providing further antibody which would convert them to antigen-antibody equilibrium or antibody excess and render them inactive.

While there is much continued enthusiasm for concepts of blocking and unblocking activities by immune complexes it should not be forgotten that immune complexes have been shown by numerous studies to have an immune depressive effect.

Other studies have provided evidence that free tumour derived antigen can by itself act in a blocking capacity (Currie and Basham, 1972; Embleton, 1973). The probability is that such antigens combine with antigen receptor sites on specifically sensitised lymphocytes and preempt the activity of these cells on tumour cell membrane located antigen (Fig. 5.1E). It can therefore be predicted that tumour cells which readily release TAA from their membranes will have a survival advantage. This has been shown to be the case in experimental tumours (Currie and Alexander, 1974) and the concept has arisen of tumours protected from effector cells by a cloud or smokescreen of released antigen (Fig. 5.1E). Free tumour antigen has been identified in animal systems and there are reports of a correlation between facility of antigen release and metastasis formation. Antigen release has also been shown to occur in human tumours (Baldwin et al., 1973; Kjaer, 1974).

If tumour associated antigens and certain classes of anti-tumour antibody form blocking factors which hamper properly tumour-restrictive functions of cell-mediated immunity, certain tentative conclusions may be drawn. These findings provide further justification (if such were needed) for surgical removal of as much tumour as possible on the grounds that a reduction in available antigen will minimise the production of blocking complexes. It is possible that a more aggressive policy will require to be adopted towards the surgical management of metastatic tumour. Radiotherapy and chemotherapy destroy large volumes of tumour *in situ* and need to be reviewed in the light of the possible effects of the relatively sudden release of large amounts of membrane and intracytoplasmic antigens from tumour cells. However it is likely that these techniques cause distortion and destruction of TAA and render them non-immunogenic. The paucity of reports of organ-specific autoimmune reactions after radiotherapy and chemotherapy suggests that antigens released after therapeutic destruction of organs and tissues are of low immunogenicity. It is also noteworthy that one of the most effective methods of immunising animals to TAA is to ligate a growing tumour and leave it *in situ*. Radiotherapy and chemotherapy depress lymphocyte numbers and function (Chapter 7) which may prevent or minimise a reaction to the antigenic material released from damaged tissues. Depressed anti-tumour antibody production, will make fewer antibody molecules available for complex formation and reduce the blocking activity. It is, in fact, possible that judicious combinations of radiotherapy and chemotherapeutic agents with selective action for different lymphocyte sub-populations may be used to "tailor" antibody production to minimise blocking activity and maximise more desirable attributes. Another approach is to remove organs such as the spleen which are the site of (blocking) antibody production but many such sites are diffuse and form parts of vital organs obviating a purely surgical approach. Splenectomy and chemotherapy or a selective immunological attack on the antibody producing cells might be effective. Plasmapheresis to remove potentially blocking antibodies may also be a useful approach. Consideration must also be given to the possibility that immune manipulation may selectively stimulate antibody synthesis and induce or strengthen blocking factors.

Attempts to reduce antibody synthesis presuppose that antibodies are always or frequently deleterious to the tumour bearer. This view can no longer be fully substantiated in the face of evidence of positive antibody activities such as target cell priming for K cell attack and inhibition of tumour cell motility (Cochran et al., 1972).

Most attention has been directed to the blocking role of complexes of tumour antigen and anti-tumour antibodies. Other types of immune complexes may occur in the sera of cancer patients and have unfavourable effects. The anti-idiotypic antibodies described by Lewis et al. (1971) are of interest in this context. They may form complexes with anti-melanoma antibodies reducing their direct tumour inhibitory activities and K cell priming functions as well as exerting some degree of immune suppression.

The great majority of studies of blocking have concerned themselves with proving and analysing the orthodox view of blocking by complete antibody molecules, tumour antigens or immune complexes. It should be remembered however that antigenic sites on tumour cells may be occluded by immuno-logically non-specific materials such as sialomucins and serum proteins and that similarly non specific materials in plasma such as macroglobulins may block effector cells (Fig. 5.1F).

An observation common to virtually all tests measuring specific and non specific functions of lymphocytes in vitro has been that serum from cancer patients will abrogate effects observed in control human serum or foetal calf serum. Blocking activity has been observed in mitogen induced transforma-tion (Han and Sokal, 1970), mixed leucocyte culture (Brooks et al., 1972), cell-mediated cytotoxicity (Hellström et al., 1969) the leucocyte migration technique (Guillou and Giles, 1973; Kjaer, 1974; Cochran et al., 1976), the leucocyte adherence inhibition assay (Halliday et al., 1974) and antigen stimulated lymphocyte blastogenesis (Vanky et al., 1975). Thus any examination of tumour-directed immunity which takes no account of the presence and role of serum factors is certainly incomplete and probably inadequate.

We recently reported a study of serum factors in melanoma patients (Cochran *et al.*, 1976) which may serve as an example of the situations described above.

Sera from 38 of 89 melanoma patients, 4 of 15 patients with other cancers and 3 of 43 control donors inhibited the migration of autologous leucocytes *in the absence of added tumour antigen* (Table 5.1). Sera from patients with clinically detectable metastatic disease and from BCG recipients were most frequently inhibitory.

Sera from 31 of 71 melanoma patients and 3 of 31 control donors increased the leucocyte migration inhibition induced by formalinised melanoma cells (Table 5.2). This activity occurred in sera from patients with all stages of malignancy, whether bearing detectable tumour or not and whether receiving BCG or not. Abrogation of tumour cell-induced leucocyte migration inhibition by serum (analogous to blocking in cytotoxicity) was less frequent, occurring with 8 of 71 melanoma patients (6 Stage III, 1 Stage I and 1 Stage II) and no control sera.

Serial studies suggest that inhibitory activity in serum correlates with active tumour growth and may antedate clinically detectable metastases by several months. The development of serum activity which increases antigen induced leucocyte migration inhibition may also predict metastases. Abrogation of antigen induced leucocyte migration inhibition is virtually confined to patients with very advanced tumour.

Studies are in progress to categorise the active components of the sera and to relate them to identified materials capable of affecting other *in vitro* techniques.

Tumour in privileged or immunologically inaccessible sites

Certain areas of the body have been held to be "privileged" in that the mediators of immune reactivity do not penetrate them. These include the eye and the tissues of the central nervous system in man and the cheek pouch in the hamster. The situation is certainly complex but tumours in these sites are at least relatively spared the attentions of the effector arm of the immune response. In Burkitt's lymphoma children often die with tumour deposits in the central nervous system which do not respond to chemotherapy despite the prior response of deposits in other sites. This may seem to indicate low responsiveness to chemotherapy, but there is evidence that at least some responses to chemotherapy in Burkitt's lymphoma involve an immunological component.

Tumours in the eye and the central nervous system are relatively seldom associated with a "reactive" infiltrate by comparison with those of the rest of

Table 5.1.

Leucocyte migration in medium supplemented with 10% autologous serum relative to migration in medium supplemented with 10% foetal calf serum. Analysis on basis of individuals and, in the case of melanoma patients by clinical stage

| Category | No. of patients | Migration in autologous serum relative to migration in foetal calf serum | | | |
| | | Inhibited[a] | | Enhanced[a] | |
		No.	%	No.	%
Melanomas	89	38	43	4	5
Stage I	17	1	6	0	0
Stage II	45	28	62	4	9
Stage III	27	9	33	0	0
Stage I and II tumour present	31	19	61	2	7
Stage I and II tumour absent	31	10	32	2	11
Stages II and III BCG recipients	36	23	64	2	6
Stages II and III No BCG	36	14	39	2	6
Other cancers	15	4	27	0	0
Control donors	43	3	7	1	2

[a]Significance assessed by the Mann Whitney Wilcoxon U test.

Table 5.2.

A comparison of leucocyte migration inhibition induced by formalinised tumour cells in medium supplemented with 10% autologous serum with that in medium containing 10% foetal calf serum. Analysis on basis of individuals and, in the case of melanoma patients, by clinical stage

| Category | No. of patients | Migration inhibition on addition of autologous serum | | | |
| | | Increased[a] | | Reduced[a] | |
		No.	%	No.	%
Melanomas	71	31	44	8	11
Stage I	12	4	33	1	8
Stage II	37	20	54	1	3
Stage III	22	7	32	6	27
Stage I and II tumour present	18	8	44	1	6
Stage I and II tumour absent	31	16	52	1	3
Stages II and III BCG recipients	23	12	52	5	22
Stages II and III No BCG	36	15	42	2	6
Control donors	31	3	10	0	0

[a]Significance assessed by the Mann Whitney Wilcoxon U test.

the body. However indices of anti-tumour immunity can be detected against tumours of privileged areas. We have found cellular and humoral immunity against ocular melanoma at a frequency similar to that observed with cutaneous melanomas (Table 5.3).

Table 5.3.

The frequency of tumour-directed cellular and humoral immunity in patients with ocular and cutaneous melanoma (Cochran—unpublished)

Patient category	Anti-tumour reactivity			
	Cellular[a]		Humoral[b]	
	$+/T$	%	$+/T$	%
Ocular melanomas	10/16	63	8/11	73
Cutaneous melanomas	80/105	76	48/83	58
Control donors	9/61	15	13/57	23

[a]Leucocyte migration inhibition by formalinised melanoma cells.
[b]Membrane immunofluorescence (patient's serum v. tissue cultured melanoma cells).

References

Baldwin, R. W., Embleton, M. J. and Price, M. R. (1973). *Int. J. Cancer* **12**, 84.
Brooks, W. H., Netsky, W. G., Normansfell, D. E. and Horwitz, D. A. (1972). *J. exp. Med.* **136**, 1631.
Brunschwig, A., Southam, C. M. and Levin, A. (1965). *Ann. Surg.* **162**, 416.
Cikes, M. (1970). *Nature* **225**, 645-647.
Cochran, A. J., Klein, E. and Kiessling, R. (1972). *J. nat. Cancer Inst.* **48**, 1657-1661.
Cochran, A. J., Thomas, C. E., Spilg, W. G. S., Grant, R. M., Cameron-Mowat, D. E., Mackie, R. M. and Lindop, G. (1973). *Yale J. Biol. Med.* **46**, 650-654.
Cochran, A. J., Mackie, R. M., Ross, C. E., Ogg, L. J. and Jackson, A. M. (1976). *Int. J. Cancer* **18**, 274.
Cremer, N. E., Taylor, D. O. and Hagens, S. J. (1966). *J. Immunol.* **96**, 495.
Currie, G. A. and Basham, C. (1972). *Brit. J. Cancer* **26**, 427-438.
Currie, G. A. and Alexander, P. (1974). *Brit. J. Cancer* **29**, 72-75.
Embleton, M. J. (1973). *Brit. J. Cancer* **28**, Suppl. 1, 142.
Essex, M., Klein, G., Snyder, S. P. and Harrold, J. B. (1971). *Int. J. Cancer* **8**, 384.
Fenyö, E. M., Klein, E., Klein, G. and Swiech, K. (1968). *J. nat. Cancer Inst.* **40**, 69-90.
Fenyö, E. M., Grundner, G., Klein, E. and Harris, H. (1971). *Exp. Cell Res.* **68**, 323.
Friberg, S. Jr., Klein, G., Wiener, F. and Harris, H. (1973). *J. nat. Cancer Inst.* **50**, 1269.
Friedman, J. M. and Fialkow, P. J. (1976). *Transplant Rev.* **28**, 17-33.
Gershon, R. K., Carter, R. L. and Kondo, K. (1967). *Nature* **213**, 674.
Guillou, P. J. and Giles, G. R. (1973). *Gut* **14**, 733.
Hakulinen, T., Houi, L., Karkinen-Kääskeläinen, M., Pentinnen, K. and Saxén, L. (1973). *Brit. med. J.* **4**, 265.

Halliday, W. J., Maluish, A. and Isbister, W. H. (1974). *Brit. J. Cancer* **29**, 31.
Han, T. and Sokal, J. E. (1970). *Amer. J. Med.* **48**, 728.
Hellström, K. E. (1959). *Transplant Bull.* **6**, 411.
Hellström, I., Hellström, K. E., Evans, C. A., Heppner, G. H., Pierce, G. E. and
    Yang, J. P. S. (1969). *Proc. nat. Acad. Sci. U.S.* **62**, 362.
Hellström, I., Hellström, K. E., Sjögren, H. O. *et al.* (1973). *Int. J. Cancer* **11**,
    116-122.
Hellström, K. E. and Hellström, I. (1974). *Clin. Immunobiol.* **2**, 233.
Kiessling, R., Klein, E. and Wigzell, H. (1975). *Europ. J. Immunol.* **5**, 112.
Kjaer, M. (1974). *Acta path. microbiol. Scand. (Sect. B)* **82**, 894.
Klein, E. and Möller, E. (1963). *J. nat. Cancer Inst.* **31**, 347.
Klein, E. and Klein, G. (1964). *J. nat. Cancer Inst.* **32**, 547.
Klein, G., Gars, U. and Harris, H. (1970). *Exp. Cell Res.* **62**, 149.
Klein, G. and Klein, E. (1976). *Transplant Proc.* (In Press.)
Laroye, G. (1973). *Lancet* **1**, 641.
Lewis, M. G., Phillips, T. M., Cook, K. B. and Blake, J. (1971). *Nature* **232**, 52-54.
Lilly, F. and Pincus, T. (1973). *Adv. Cancer Res.* **17**, 231.
Malmgren, R. A., Bennison, B. E. and McKinley, T. L. S. (1952). *Proc. Soc. exp.
    Biol. Med.* **79**, 484.
Möller, E. and Möller, G. (1962). *J. exp. Med.* **127**, 523.
Muhlbock, O. and Dux, A. (1974). *J. nat. Cancer Inst.* **53**, 993.
Mukojima, T., Gunven, P. and Klein, G. (1973). *J. nat. Cancer Inst.* **51**, 1319-1321.
Old, L. J., Boyse, E. A., Clarke, D. A. and Carswell, E. A. (1962). *Ann. N.Y. Acad.
    Sci.* **101**, 80.
Peterson, R. D. A., Hendrickson, R. and Good, R. A. (1963). *Proc. Soc. exp. Biol.
    Med.* **114**, 517.
Prehn, R. T. (1976). *Transplant Rev.* **28**, 34-42.
Sjögren, H. O., Hellström, I. and Bansal, S. C. (1971). *Proc. nat. Acad. Sci. U.S.*
    68, 1372-1375.
Stewart, A. M., Webb, J. and Hewitt, D. (1958). *Brit. med. J.* **1**, 1495.
Stjernswärd, J. (1969). *Antibiotica Chemotherap.* **15**, 213.
Tevethia, S. S., McMillan, V. L., Kaplan, P. M. and Bushong, S. C. (1971).
    J. Immunol. **106**, 1295.
Vanky, F., Trempe, G., Klein, E. and Stjernswärd, J. (1975). *Int. J. Cancer* **16**, 113.
Yefenof, E. and Klein, G. (1974). *Exp. Cell Res.* **88**, 217.

6

Practical Applications of Studies of the Immunology of Cancer Patients

---

The techniques of clinical immunology have been used to investigate cancer patients in four major ways. Attempts have been made to examine the immunological integrity (immunocompetence) of patients at cancer diagnosis, during therapy and as the disease progresses. Immunological techniques have been assessed as methods of diagnosing cancer, both prior to the development of clinically evident disease and when overt tumour is present, but before its exact nature is ascertained. An area of interest and promise is the serial examination of materials from cancer patients after therapy in an attempt to predict the development of metastatic or recurrent tumour. Attempts have been made to relate immunocompetence and tumour-directed immunity to prognosis.

General Assessment of the Immunological Competence of Cancer Patients

The significance of this type of assessment depends on the assumption that patients develop cancer, or that their cancers grow and spread because of immunological defects. Immunological abnormalities are detectable in cancer patients, but are not uniform and tend to occur later in the disease rather than earlier, suggesting that they are a result of the cancer rather than its cause. We cannot, however, exclude the existence of inherent selective defects in immune recognition or function which may permit tumour development and progression in some patients. Two types of immunological defect must therefore be considered; a limited defect present at and possibly before the earliest stages of tumour development and a more crass defect which occurs in parallel with the failure of other body systems late in the disease. Additionally the timing and nature of the defects varies between tumours of the reticuloendothelial system and those arising in other organs. This is hardly surprising as tumours affecting specialised organs often reduce or distort their function, and it is in this light that immunological abnormalities in the leukaemias and lymphomas must be viewed. While the naive concept of the cancer patient as an immunological cripple *ab initio* cannot be substantiated, studies of general and specific immunological functions remain important and seem likely to aid the planning of therapy and may increase accuracy in prognostication.

An extensive array of tests is available for this type of examination. Broadly they permit the assessment of the integrity of the various components of the immunological apparatus. They allow assessment of the extent to which memory of previous episodes of immunological stimulation is retained and the nature, quality and completeness of responses to new antigens which the individual has not previously encountered.

Studies of Reactions *in vivo*

SKIN TESTS WITH RECALL ANTIGENS

These employ the intradermal injection of small quantities of semi-purified antigens from widespread bacteria, viruses and fungi with which a majority of individuals will have had contact and to which many may reasonably be expected to have developed sensitisation. This response is indicated by a delayed cutaneous skin reaction to the intradermal injection of the appropriate antigen; the development 24 to 48 hours after introduction of the antigen of a palpable measurable raised area at the injection site with or without attendant oedema and erythema. Histological examination of the reaction site shows infiltration with lymphocytes and macrophages, perivascular in the early stages of the reaction, but more diffusely distributed later. There may also be variable vascular congestion and oedema and a few polymorphonuclear granulocytes may be present. The reaction is best exemplified clinically and histologically by the classical tuberculin reaction.

The allergens most commonly used are extracts of *Mycobacterium tuberculosis* such as old tuberculin, extracts of *Candida*, of *Trichophyton rubrum*, of the *mumps* virus and of the *Streptococcus*, usually streptokinase-streptodornase (Varidase). In the selection of appropriate antigens due attention should be paid to local disease patterns and practices in relation to prophylaxis. For instance the tuberculin reaction is widely used in Great Britain and a high proportion of the normal population show skin reactivity in this test. This reflects the high incidence of tuberculosis which existed when the older segment of the population was young and the widespread use of immunisation with *Bacillus Calmette-Guérin* adopted in the 1950s and practised since then. The situation in the United States of America is different with a relatively low level of endemic tuberculosis and the very limited use of BCG immunoprophylaxis. The most sensible policy in selecting a panel of recall antigens is to examine a range of normal individuals against numerous antigens and to choose a test panel of antigens on the basis of their pattern of reactivity.

Studies of recall antigen reactivity of cancer patients are relatively numerous (Lamb *et al.*, 1962; Solowey and Rapaport, 1965; Eilber and Morton, 1970; Wells *et al.*, 1973; Rosato *et al.*, 1974) and although they have yielded somewhat conflicting results when the results of individual antigens are considered, there appears to be a general consensus that patients with early cancer have no major deficit of immunological memory as assessed by recall antigen skin tests, but that a decline of this type of reactivity occurs in patients with advanced disease (Eilber and Morton, 1970) those with metastatic disease (Solowey and Rapaport, 1965) and those showing debilitation (Lamb *et al.*, 1962). Our own experience conforms well with this view and in a recent study (Cochran *et al.*, 1976) we found no difference in a comparison of a group of cancer patients and control donors but a reduced frequency of reactions to *Candida DHS* and Varidase in patients with metastatic disease when compared with individuals who had early cancer. Patients with metastases generally reacted to fewer antigens of the test panel (Table 6.1).

The fact that recall skin test reactivity is normal in early cancer and low when the disease is advanced suggests that a decrease in this component of the immune response has little to do with the development of malignant disease and that the later decline is a sequel of disease progression rather than causally associated with metastasis formation. Nonetheless serial testing with a standard group of skin test antigens might predict metastases although interpretation is complicated by the possibility that repeated antigenic stimulation, even with the tiny doses of antigens employed in skin testing, may induce specific immunisation or reimmunisation.

The mechanisms of the stage-related decline in skin test reactivity is poorly understood. It is generally believed, on the basis of very little evidence, to be part of a general depression of immune reactivity. However more specific defects of antigen recognition and mobilisation may be involved and Amos *et al.* (1965) raised the interesting possibility that a decline in the incidence of "passenger" lymphocytes in the skin may be significant.

SKIN TESTS WITH NEW ANTIGENS

If tumour cells develop completely new antigens or re-express antigens not normally exposed during adult life the capacity to mount new immune

Table 6.1.

Recall antigen skin tests in cancer patients and controls

	SKIN TEST ANTIGENS										Positive Versus	
	Mantoux		Mumps		Candida DHS		T rubrum		Varidase		0-2	3-5
	+/T	%	+/T	%	+/T	%	+/T	%	+/T	%		
Cancer patients	40/60	67	27/50	54	19/25	76	8/48	17	53/60	88	24/52 (46%)	28/52 (54%)
No metastases	17/22	77	14/24	58	8/8	100 ⎤ᵃ	2/18	11	21/31	100 ⎤ᵇ	9/23 (39%)	14/23 (61%)
Metastases	21/33	64	13/26	50	5/14	35 ⎦	6/30	20	25/33	76 ⎦	11/20 (55%)	9/20 (45%)
Control donors	36/48	75	6/20	30	16/20	80	6/48	13	40/48	83	19/42 (45%)	23/42 (55%)

[a]Difference significant p <0.01.
[b]Difference significant p <0.02.

responses is clearly critical. Studies of this type seem likely to be more relevant than the auditing of memory function by recall antigen challenge. Recent studies have examined the capacity of cancer patients to respond to novel antigens, antigens to which the normal population would not be expected to show sensitisation. The agents employed have been synthetic contact sensitising agents such as dinitrochlorobenzene (DNCB) (Epstein and Kligman, 1959; Eilber and Morton, 1970; Chakravorty *et al.*, 1973) or the closely related dinitrofluorobenzene (DNFB) (Levin *et al.*, 1964) or biological molecules such as keyhole limpet haemocyanin (Swanson and Schwartz, 1967), horseshoe crab haemocyanin (Bandilla *et al.*, 1969), bacteriophage øX174 (Uhr *et al.*, 1962) and α-haemocyanin of *Helix pomatia* (deGast, 1975).

Primary antigens induce an immune response in virtually all normal individuals. In cancer patients they are claimed either to induce a reaction in a lower proportion of individuals (Levin *et al.*, 1964; Krant *et al.*, 1968) or a weaker response (deGast, 1975). The role of primary antigen testing in prognostication and monitoring is discussed below. Repeated testing, however, may lead to re-immunisation, complicating interpretation, a problem which may be avoided by employing *in vitro* assays (Miller and Levis, 1973; Hamilton *et al.*, 1976).

Primary antigens thus offer some assistance in the assessment of immuno-competence. Considerable care is necessary in their use as agents such as DNCB and DNFB may cause considerable irritation and even extensive skin necrosis and viral contamination of the biological agents is possible.

An alternative approach to assessing the ability to mount a new immune response would be to examine the capacity to reject allografted skin. The technology and interpretation of skin grafting is however considerably more cumbersome and demanding than that of sensitisation and challenge with primary antigens, which makes homografting a less attractive means of assessing immunological integrity.

The Assessment of Immunological Integrity by *in vitro* Techniques

This approach has the considerable advantage of relative technical simplicity, but the techniques suffer from the handicap that they assess isolated components of a sophisticated process which depends on subtle interactions of many different cell types and complex molecules for its effectiveness. Results obtained in this way are highly artificial and interpretation of even grossly abnormal results remains largely a matter of speculation. Severe distortions of normal values observed *in vitro* are often not associated with increased susceptibility to infection suggesting considerable reserve capacity in these systems.

ASSESSMENT OF LYMPHOCYTE NUMBERS, SUBPOPULATIONS AND NON-SPECIFIC FUNCTIONS

Quantification of lymphocytes in the peripheral blood

The assessment of lymphocyte numbers and their proportion as part of a differential white count is such a simple process that it would be undesirable to ignore information obtainable in this manner. Most studies of lymphocyte numbers have not, however, found a significant variation between cancer patients and control populations nor have they demonstrated differences in the lymphocyte count with variations in cancer stage in patients not receiving radiotherapy or chemotherapy. This has certainly been our own experience (Table 6.2—Cochran et al., 1976). Simple counting of lymphocytes remains

Table 6.2.

Lymphocyte counts in cancer patients and controls

		Lymphocytes/cu. mm.	
	No.	mean ± SEM[a]	range
Cancer patients	92	2047 ± 81	440-4400
No metastases	60	2088 ± 114	550-4400
Metastases	22	1784 ± 139	440-3560
Control donors	97	2100 ± 71	550-3970

[a]Standard error of the mean.

an important part of the haematological evaluation of cancer patients, but appears to have a very limited place in immunological assessment. A further simple examination of lymphocytes is to estimate the proportion of small, medium and large lymphocytes and plasma cells in the peripheral blood. Crowther et al. (1969) found an increase in medium sized and large lymphocytes in patients with Hodgkin's disease and also observed occasional circulating plasma cells. Similar changes occur in conditions of known antigenic challenge such as infections, after immunisation and in autoimmune disease and this rather neglected approach may be worthy of further investigation.

Lymphocyte subpopulations

Simple morphological assessment of lymphocytes has been overtaken by the realisation that light microscopically similar lymphocytes can be subgrouped on the basis of their membrane characteristics. The initial subdivision was into thymus dependent (T) cells and thymus independent (B) cells by analogy with the situation in animals and fowls and on the basis of studies of immune deficiency disorders in animals and man (Roitt *et al.*, 1969). From a functional standpoint these populations are distinct, the T cells being those actually or potentially concerned with cell-mediated immunity and the B cells being concerned in humoral immunity and including the precursors of antibody synthesising plasma cells. The study of lymphocyte subpopulations in man has proceeded by the exploitation of membrane characteristics specific for the different subpopulations. T lymphocytes aggregate the erythrocytes of different species to form rosette shaped clusters (E-rosettes) (Fig. 6.1), the chicken erythrocyte being that most used in practice, and are virtually non-reactive with fluorescein-labelled anti-Ig sera. B cells react with anti-Ig sera and thus have Ig molecules incorporated in their membranes. B cells also form rosettes, but with IgM antibody primed erythrocytes in the presence of complement (EAC rosettes). This reflects the presence of receptors for the Fc part of the Ig molecule and for the third component of complement. It is also possible to demonstrate Fc receptors on some cells by their capacity to bind heterologous erythrocytes coated with IgG antibody (EA rosettes) or fluorescein labelled, heat aggregated IgG. As other cells, including monocytes and polymorphs, bear Fc and complement receptors the EAC and EA rosette technique can no longer be regarded as specific for B cells, except in exhaustively purified lymphocyte populations. On the basis of E and EAC rosetting techniques and membrane-associated Ig it was initially held that about 70% of human peripheral blood lymphocytes were T cells and 30% B cells. Some workers, however, found a proportion of lymphocytes to be neither T nor B cells ("null" cells) and others observed some lymphocytes to have characteristics of both T and B lineage. The function of null cells is unclear but they may be precursor cells, uncommitted to T or B allegiance and function. The function of cells showing mixed T and B cell characteristics is not known.

Other techniques claimed to assist in the characterisation of T and B lymphocytes are electron microscopy and the capacity to respond to various antigens and mitogenic substances by blast transformation (see below).

Recent reports suggest subgroups of T cells including "active" T cells (Wybran and Fudenberg, 1973), T cells capable of forming E-rosettes under suboptimal conditions, "autorosetting" T cells which form E-type rosettes with autologous erythrocytes and may be antigenically activated lymphocytes and "super rosetting" T cells which form rosettes with more than six erythrocytes. Interest has also focused on mononuclear cells capable of killing target cells primed with antibody (K-cells). Monocytes can certainly do this but in ultra-pure lymphocyte preparations a population exists which functions in the manner of K cells (Chapter 3). The situation reflects the evolutionary stage of classification, with a steadily increasing number of classes of lymphocytes, many characterised by seemingly illogical technology.

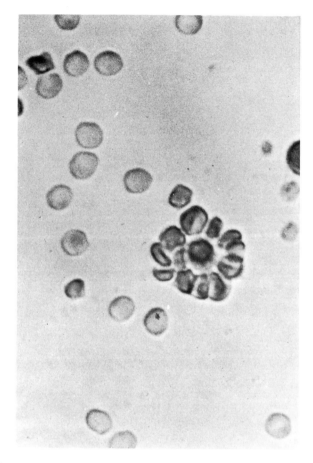

Fig. 6.1. An "E" rosette showing a lymphocyte with aggregated erythrocytes.
Photograph by courtesy of Dr. G. P. Sandilands.

The important fact remains that lymphocytes are heterogeneous and analysis of this heterogeneity is likely to provide a better understanding of the immunological apparatus.

There has inevitably been interest in the possibility of variations in lymphocyte subpopulations in malignant disease. Two major possibilities exist. There may be a gross reduction in the number of T or B cells present, which may lead to impairment of the immunological apparatus, or there may be no numerical decrease in one or other type of lymphocyte, in which case the problem becomes one of identifying functional derangements of the lymphocytes. The results point to relatively minor variations in the classical T and B cell population (Nemoto *et al.*, 1974; Gross *et al.*, 1975; Dellon *et al.*, 1975; Stein *et al.*, 1976; Kopersztych *et al.*, 1976; Wilkins and Olkowski, 1977). We found the frequency of T and B lymphocytes similar in a comparison of a group of cancer patients and controls (Cochran *et al.*, 1976) and this accords well with several other studies of cancer patients who had not received radiotherapy or chemotherapy. However some patients had a very low T cell count suggesting that while in *most* patients the cause of T cell inefficiency had to be sought in perverted function, a few suffer from an absolute reduction in the number of T cells. It is of course also possible that even these residual lymphocytes are functionally subnormal. Fc receptor +ve cells were significantly increased in patients with metastatic disease. Variations in lymphocyte subpopulations have been observed. Wybran and Fudenberg (1973) and Claudy *et al.* (1976) recorded a decrease in "active" T cells in melanoma patients, while we (Cochran *et al.*, 1976) found an increase in "active" T cells (assessed by a technique slightly different from that of Wybran), autorosetting T cells and super-rosetting T cells in melanoma patients (Table 6.3).

The significant observation is that subpopulations of lymphocytes do appear to vary in a detectable fashion in malignant disease. The technology of assessing such subpopulations remains difficult and cumbersome, and accurate definitive elucidation of these variations and of their significance must probably await considerable simplification of the techniques employed to delineate them.

Mitogen induced lymphocyte blastogenesis

On confrontation with an antigen lymphocytes undergoing sensitisation or presensitised lymphocytes being restimulated undergo the complex series of changes which lead to mitosis, changes which may be detected by an increase in size of the cells involved or an increase in the incorporation of radiolabelled aminoacids. Specific antigen-driven blast transformation has been discussed in Chapter 3. Other materials (mitogens) which are not antigens in the proper sense of the word can also cause lymphocyte blast transformation, in a manner which is not immunologically specific, but which provides a measure of cellular activities which are important as the generation of immunity requires lymphocytes to replicate rapidly. The most commonly used mitogens have been phytohaemagglutinin (PHA), Pokeweed mitogen (PWM) and Concanavalin-A. Different mitogens are variably active against T and B lymphocytes and provide a further means of dissecting these subpopulations. Table 6.4 summarises the mitogen responsiveness of T and B cells.

The technology of these tests is deceptively simple and some of the very extensive literature on lymphocyte blastogenesis, is of rather doubtful quality. In these techniques, no less than in any other, attention to detail

Table 6.3.

Lymphocyte subpopulations in melanoma patients and controls

	T cells			FC +ve cells			Active T cells			Autorosetting T cells			Super rosetting T cells		
	No.	$m \pm$ SEM[a]	range	No.	$m^b \pm$ SEM	range	No.	$m^c \pm$ SEM	range	No.	$m^c \pm$ SEM	range	No.	$m^c \pm$ SEM	range
Cancer patients	28	72 ± 2	49-88	28	29 ± 2	8-47	28	83 ± 3	35-100	28	7 ± 1	1-23	28	77 ± 3	43-99
No metastases	7	70 ± 4	49-81	7	21 ± 3	8-27	7	89 ± 6	69-100	7	7 ± 2	2-10	7	69 ± 2	42-90
Metastases	21	72 ± 2	55-88	21	32 ± 2	20-52	21	81 ± 3	34-98	21	8 ± 2	1-23	21	81 ± 2	67-98
Control donors	50	73 ± 1	55-83	50	28 ± 1	15-45	50	72 ± 3	35-100	50	4 ± 1	1-20	50	66 ± 3	30-95

[a]Standard error of the mean.
[b]Percentage of total lymphocytes.
[c]Percentage of total T lymphocytes.

Table 6.4.

The mitogen responsiveness of lymphocyte subpopulations

Mitogen	Responsive lymphocyte population	Comment
Concanavalin-A	T	
Phytohaemagglutinin	T	may also act on B lymphocyte
E. coli lipopolysaccharide	B	
Pneumococcal polysaccharide	B	
Anti-human F (ab¹)₂ serum	B	
Pokeweed mitogen	T and B	
Purified protein derivative of tuberculin	T	in pre-sensitised subjects
	B	in non-presensitised subjects

and the inclusion of full controls is vital and the use of dose response curves desirable. It is not possible for a technician to perform occasional transformations and produce high quality data of low variability. This would seem self-evident and yet the literature on transformation studies in cancer patients is often self-contradicting and ridden with paradoxes, at least some of which may be attributed to technical factors.

The situation is made even more complicated by the fact that lymphocyte transformation may be reduced by an intrinsic defect of lymphocytes or by materials circulating in the plasma which depress inherently normal lymphocytes (Humphrey et al., 1975).

Some authors have found reduced mitogen induced lymphocyte blastogenesis in malignant disease (Whittaker et al., 1971; Catalona et al. 1973; Hersh and Oppenheim, 1965; Knight and Davidson, 1975) while others (Nelson, 1969; Roberts, 1970; Sample et al., 1971; Paty and Bone, 1973; Golub et al., 1974) including ourselves (Table 6.5) have not. The situation may differ for different malignancies, lymphomas with their special relationship to the cells of the immune apparatus being different from non-lymphoid malignancies.

In vitro reactions to non-tumour antigens

The problems of serial skin tests with recall antigens could be overcome by *in vitro* studies of the memory capacity. Tuberculoprotein can be used for this purpose in populations where tuberculin reactivity is the rule. Where this is not the case the local population will generally be reactive to other antigens such as brucellin or fungal materials and identification of a locally relevant alternative to tuberculoprotein will permit the application of this approach.

As the majority of Scots are tuberculin positive we examined PPD induced transformation in study groups assessed for PHA transformation (Table 6.5) but found no significant differences in mean PPD transformation indices in comparisons of cancer patients and controls and of cancer patients with and without metastases. This approach is not ideal as the transformation indices induced by PPD are relatively small, and different populations of lymphocytes respond in sensitised and non-sensitised individuals (Table 6.4).

Table 6.5.

Studies of lymphocyte transformation in cancer patients and controls

	PHA			PPD		
	No.	Mean[a] ± SEM[b]	range	No.	Mean ± SEM	range
Cancer patients	52	53 ± 8	3-200	19	3·2 ± 1	1-15
No metastases	25	50 ± 9	4-166	7	3·4 ± 1·8	1-14
Metastases	13	61 ± 16	3-200	7	3·4 ± 1·8	1-15
Controls	39	37 ± 9	3-270	34	2·2 ± 0·3	1-9

[a]Uptake of tritiated thymidine in mitogen stimulated cultures (mean of 3 observations)

   Uptake of tritiated thymidine in unstimulated cultures (mean of 3 observations)

[b]Standard error of the mean.

We have therefore turned to examining tuberculoprotein sensitisation by a leucocyte migration assay. As PPD is difficult to handle in this technique we are at present examining the effect of BCG on leucocyte migration. This appears to offer some advantages over PPD induced lymphocyte transformation. A positive reaction indicates the existence of an intact antigen recognition system and also demonstrates the ability to produce at least one lymphokine. A logistic advantage is that by this method results are available within 24 hours compared to the 4-5 days required for transformation studies. This study is incomplete at the time of writing. Preliminary results indicate that it is necessary to perform a dose-response study of each individual and that many cancer patients only react to relatively high concentrations of BCG while age matched disease free controls react to much lower concentrations.

Mixed lymphocyte culture (MLC)
This seems a potentially useful technique. An intact reaction in MLC is likely to indicate the persistence of the all important capacity to recognise a new antigen as foreign and to mount a cellular immune reaction to it. This is thus an *in vitro* equivalent of sensitisation and challenge with new antigens

such as DNCB but excludes the morbidity associated with such *in vivo* procedures. Golub *et al*. (1974) found that anomalies of MLC and mitogen-induced transformation may occur separately in cancer patients, suggesting that separate deficiencies of antigen recognition and lymphocyte proliferative capacity may exist. It is clear that the two activities need not be closely linked and MLC is thus a useful parallel of mitogen transformation and not merely a variant of the latter type of approach. In addition to the above report depressed MLC reactivity has been recorded in cancer patients by other groups (Han and Takita, 1972; Sucia-Foca *et al*., 1973), and related to the presence of inhibitory factors in the patient's serum.

Capacity to produce lymphokines

T lymphocytes (and possibly to a lesser degree and in special circumstances B lymphocytes) confronted with an antigen to which they are sensitised release a variety of non-immunoglobulin substances known collectively as lymphokines or lymphocyte activation products. To date about twenty such substances have been identified and named pragmatically for the effects they produce in the *in vitro* systems used to detect them. The best known include macrophage and/or leucocyte migration inhibition factor, macrophage aggregation factor, macrophage chemotactic factor, blastogenic factor, interferon and a lymphotoxic factor. The precise relationship of these different factors to each other and their biological role *in vivo* remain to be elucidated but their production is an important index of the functional integrity of lymphocytes. The technology of generation of these factors is relatively simple, involving the cultivation of lymphocytes with an antigen to which the lymphocyte donor is known to be sensitised and the subsequent testing of the harvested culture supernatants in an appropriate assay system. Lymphokines may also be generated by mitogen stimulated lymphocytes. Quantification of lymphokines would also seem technically feasible. There is considerable current interest in this type of assessment of lymphocyte function and its wider use in the assessment of immunological competence seems certain.

ASSESSMENT OF THE ACTIVITY OF OTHER RELEVANT CELL POPULATIONS

Macrophages

The bone marrow derived cells of the "mononuclear phagocytic system", blood monocytes, tissue macrophages, Kupffer cells and so on, have been regarded as primarily important for their endocytic activity; the phagocytosis of soluble and insoluble particles and the destruction of ingested materials by lysosomal enzymic hydrolysis. More recently it has been recognised that they have an importance in the immune response. In the afferent arc they ingest and process antigen, presenting a highly immunogenic complex of antigenic fragments and macrophage ribonucleoprotein to the lymphocytes. They also cooperate with T and B lymphocytes to produce an enhanced immune response. Lymphocytes in their turn influence macrophages by their products, including migration inhibition factor, macrophage spreading factor, specific macrophage arming factor (Evans and Alexander, 1972) and a cytophilic T cell derived material which makes macrophages more receptive to antigen (Feldman, 1969). In the efferent arc macrophages *per se* have been shown to be specifically and nonspecifically cytostatic and cytotoxic to target cells including tumour cells and produce a specific macrophage cytotoxin (McIvor and Weiser, 1971). They also enhance lymphocyte mediated cell killing (Lonai and Feldman, 1971) and kill antibody primed target cells (Fakhri *et al.*, 1973; Allison, 1972).

In a complete assessment of the immunology of a cancer patient consideration should therefore be given to the functional integrity of this important group of cells. Morphological and enzyme histochemical techniques should permit the enumeration of macrophages in mixed populations of cells, although the satisfactory separation of macrophages in good condition from solid tissues, such as tumours, remains technically difficult. Well established methods exist for the assessment of macrophage phagocytosis, chemotaxis, motility and responsiveness to migration inhibition factor. Established techniques also exist for the assessment of specific and non-specific macrophage cytotoxicity (see Lejeune, 1975 for review). The assessment of macrophage performance in antigen handling and cellular cooperation and the investigation of macrophage products remains at a developmental stage and the techniques employed are not yet applicable in a routine screening role.

Despite the useful technology available studies of macrophage function in cancer remain disproportionately few. This is no doubt largely due to the concentration of effort on the lymphocyte in recent years and it seems highly desirable and probable that this imbalance is in process of correction.

Polymorphonuclear leucocytes

While not a component of the classic immune response, these cells as prime movers in the acute inflammatory response are worthy of consideration in any assessment of the integrity of the cancer patients' cellular defence mechanisms. A variety of *in vitro* tests are available to assess their function. These include tests of phagocytic activity, tests of bactericidal capacity, an assessment of the integrity of the hexose monophosphate shunt of resting and stimulated granulocytes (Keusch *et al.*, 1972) and the examination of their ability to take up and reduce the nitroblue tetrazolium dye (NBT) (Park *et al.*, 1968). All are technically demanding, partly because of the difficulty of handling these inherently fragile cells. The results of the application of these tests have to date been rather varied. Granulocyte phagocytic activity has been reported by some authors to be reduced in acute myeloid leukaemia (Rosner et al., 1970; Strauss et al., 1970; Cline, 1973) and acute lymphoblastic leukaemia (Rosner et al., 1970; Strauss et al., 1970) although normal values were found in acute myeloid leukaemia by others (Silver et al., 1957). Leucocyte bactericidal capacity has generally been found to be reduced in leukaemia patients (Baude et al., 1954; Groch et al., 1965; Karlinske and Hoeprich, 1969). NBT uptake was found to be below normal in the unstimulated leucocytes of patients with acute lymphoblastic leukaemia by Pickering et al. (1975) but this finding is in contrast to normal levels found in patients with lymphomas (Ashburn et al., 1973), chronic myeloid leukaemia (Tan et al., 1973), acute leukaemias (Miller and Kaplan, 1970) and neuroblastoma (Silver et al., 1957). In acute leukaemias hexose monophosphate shunt activity was found to be increased in resting leucocytes and decreased in stimulated leucocytes (Skeel et al., 1971; Pickering et al., 1975) but normal levels were found in acute leukaemic patients receiving radiotherapy (Baehner et al., 1973).

Clearly much remains to be done in this area, which like the macrophage studies has been overshadowed by recent concentration on the role and functions of the lymphocyte.

ASSESSMENT OF HUMORAL FACTORS

Quantification of serum immunoglobulin levels

One of the most readily assessed immunological parameters is the level of immunoglobulin (Ig) in the peripheral blood, usually by single radial immunodiffusion (Mancini et al., 1965) against calibrated standards. Unaltered levels of Ig suggest that B lymphocytes are present in reasonably normal numbers and that B lymphocyte based Ig biosynthetic pathways are functioning normally.

There are many reports of variations in serum Ig levels in cancer patients (Fahey, 1965; Bernier, 1964; Roberts et al., 1973; Barkas et al., 1976) including increased IgA in oral cancer (Mandel et al., 1973), prostatic cancer (Ablin et al., 1972), carcinoma of the cervix uteri (Plesnicar, 1972) and nasopharyngeal carcinoma (Wara et al., 1975). In a study of breast cancer and malignant melanoma we (Cochran et al., 1976) found significantly raised IgG and IgA in cancer patients sera but normal levels of IgM. We could detect no difference between patients with primary cancer and those with metastases (Table 6.6), in contrast to Smith (1972) and Waldmann et al. (1972) who found Ig to decline in patients with advanced cancer.

An increase of IgM antibody would fit best with a primary immune response, however even if this is the case there is no proof that the stimulating

Table 6.6.

Serum Ig levels in cancer patients and controls

	N	IgG		IgA		IgM	
		$\overline{M} \pm$ SEM	range	$\overline{M} \pm$ SEM	ramge	$\overline{M} \pm$ SEM	range
Cancer patients	91	1163[a,b] ± 46	385-2675	305[c] ± 30	75-2460	157 ± 8	47-548
No metastases	56	1196 ± 68	460-2275	297 ± 27	75-920	155 ± 10	47-324
Metastases	24	1163 ± 103	385-2675	342 ± 96	80-2460	165 ± 21	86-548
Controls	107	904[b] ± 29	470-2160	215[c] ± 12	3-672	145 ± 8	49-366

[a]mg/100 ml.
[b]Comparison of these two values shows a very highly significant difference, $p < 0.001$.
[c]Comparison of these two values shows a highly significant difference, $p < 0.01$.

antigens are tumour neoantigens, it being entirely possible that the response is to antigens of micro-organisms causing intercurrent infection. By the time a tumour is clinically apparent the body has been exposed to its neoantigens for a long period (though new antigens may continually emerge during tumour growth) in which case antibodies are likely to be IgG.

The problem is not the detection of abnormalities of immunoglobulin levels, but the interpretation of such anomalies as are observed. The immunoglobulin fraction of the plasma proteins includes molecules with and without antibody specificity. The proportion of molecules with antibody specificity which are reactive with tumour associated antigens is impossible to assess but is probably rather small. Patients with advanced cancer are prone to infections, a tendency which may be exacerbated by immuno-suppressive treatment and alterations in serum proteins may be a consequence of this rather than a direct result of the cancer. Again patients who are unable to eat or retain food as a result of their disease or its treatment may develop malnutrition which will be reflected in the plasma proteins. It is difficult to see how Ig estimations may be useful in the assessment and monitoring of cancer patients.

Assessment of complement activation and quantification of individual complement components

If tumour associated antigens do induce an immune response it is likely that their interaction with some of the antibodies produced will activate the complement system and lead to consumption of complement components. Techniques exist for the quantification of the individual components of complement [for instance, Kent and Fife (1963), Laurel (1965), Thompson and Lachmann (1970) and immunodiffusion for C1q, C3, C4, C7 and C3 proactivator employing commercially available plates] which permit a relatively exact assessment of this system.

Some authors have recorded a raised level of complement in cancer patients (McKenzie *et al.*, 1967; Meier and Grob, 1972; Verhaegen *et al.*, 1976) while others have found average values in cancer patients similar to those in normal individuals, but a wider variation in individual values in cancer patients (Southam and Goldsmith, 1951; Southam and Siegel, 1966; Chang, 1967; Inai *et al.*, 1967). Verhaegen *et al.* found normal levels in patients in remission and that complement levels increased with advancing disease but declined terminally. This sequence of events is similar to that observed with experimental carcinomas in rabbits by Yoshida and Ito (1968).

We recently examined 31 cancer patients and found abnormalities of individual components of complement in 16 (51%) (Cochran *et al.*, 1976). No such abnormalities were found in a parallel simultaneous examination of 70 normal individuals. No single abnormality was characteristic of the cancer patients, anomalies being found in C1q, C3, C5,6 and C7. The problem once again is one of interpretation. While the observed abnormalities *may* indicate a continuing TAA-anti TAA immune reaction, other factors such as intercurrent infection, including the activation of the alternative pathway by endotoxin and the effects of tumour necrosis may be involved. Another justification for studying complement is that in individuals with congenital or acquired anomalies of synthesis or interaction of the subcomponents of complement, the activities of complement dependent antibody will be reduced or abolished which may have a deleterious effect on antitumour immune activities. For the present complement anomalies in cancer patients, while worthy of continued evaluation, must remain of unproven value in assessment or monitoring.

Circulating immune complexes
The existence of a continuing reaction between TAA and antibodies to them would be expected to produce circulating immune complexes. Categorisation of serum factors which abrogate tumour directed cell-mediated cytostasis and cytotoxicity confirms that such complexes exist and that their presence correlates with tumour activity (Chapter 5). Immune complexes have also been shown to cause nephrotic syndrome in a variety of human malignancies and the evidence is that they are complexes of TAA-anti-TAA (Lee *et al.*, 1966; Loughbridge and Lewis, 1971; Plager and Stutzman, 1971).

As the techniques employed in detecting reaction-abrogating blocking factors are complicated and technically demanding there is a strong argument for attempting to detect immune complexes by (relatively) simpler tests which rely on the physico-chemical properties of such complexes. Unfortunately the technology for this type of assessment remains distinctly limited. In a preliminary study (Cochran *et al.*, 1976) we sought complexes by looking for anti-complementary activity (Mayer, 1961) in the sera of 12 melanoma patients and 22 normal individuals; finding such activity in only two sera, both from melanoma patients. Currently evolving techniques such as the effect of serum on the number of Fc positive lymphocytes (Jewell and McLennan, 1973), C1q deviation from artificial complexes by serum (Sobel *et al.*, 1975), the effect of serum on antibody dependent cell-mediated cytotoxicity (Barkas *et al.*, 1976) and the effect of autologous serum on leucocyte migration in the absence of added antigen (Cochran *et al.*, 1976) may make this type of assessment simpler.

Assessment of titres of natural antibodies and of antibodies to neoantigens or common infective agents
While various studies of this type exist, identifiable reductions of antibodies would require a major degree of immune depression which would be more readily identified by other techniques *in vivo* and *in vitro*.

A more sophisticated approach is to challenge patients with neoantigens or with bacterial antigens and examine the development of a new antibody response or the enhancement of an existing one (Lytton *et al.*, 1964; Hughes and McKay, 1965).

In any search for reduced immunocompetence it is necessary to consider the existence of influences known to depress reticuloendothelial functions such as drugs, malnutrition, carcinogens and materials produced by tumour cells (Snyderman *et al.*, 1976; Otu *et al.*, 1977). This topic is discussed in detail in Chapter 7.

Cancer Diagnosis by Immunological Techniques

In a majority of patients the diagnosis of malignancy is all too readily made on clinical history and examination supplemented by radiology, scintigraphy and histology or cytology. However, in some individuals the diagnosis is obscure or the primary site or nature of the malignancy remains indeterminate and additional evidence from immunological or immunochemical tests would be valuable. Such tests would also permit the rapid and repeated screening of populations with premalignant conditions or those known to have a higher than average risk of developing cancer, such as cigarette smokers and asbestos workers. Tests of this kind, requiring neither anaesthetic nor surgical operation would be virtually free of morbidity. They are also attractive from a logistic and economic standpoint as they need not involve medical personnel other than in the taking of samples for analysis.

Sadly, with a few notable exceptions, this glittering prospect remains just that. However, we know very precisely the requirements for tests of this nature.

(i) The materials should be produced by, or induced by, or selectively associated with tumour cells.

(ii) They should be exclusive to tumour cells, but a major quantitative difference between tumours and other tissues would be acceptable from a practical standpoint.

(iii) The materials must be accessible. They should not be sequestered in or on the tumour cells and ideally would readily be detected in blood and urine.

(iv) They should reflect the number of tumour cells present and rapidly equilibrate with increases or decreases in tumour volume.

(v) They should be detectable by relatively simple techniques which do not require expensive sophisticated apparatus and which permit the rapid performance of large numbers of tests by technically trained personnel. As an alternative, tests should be capable of being automated.

Two broad groups of materials are currently candidates for use in cancer diagnosis: products synthesised by tumour cells and the indices of immune reactions to tumour associated antigens.

TUMOUR PRODUCTS (MARKERS)

These are by no means all immunological in the classical sense of being auto-immunogenic but most are immunogenic in experimental animals and diagnostic antisera can be raised against them. This is one of the few real success stories of recent years, but specific tumour products have been identified for relatively few tumours. If markers can be found for most or all cancers, immunodiagnosis of malignancy will be a practical proposition. This statement, however, has to be interpreted cautiously since as well as identifying products for each tumour, it is essential to show that they are specific for the tumour. Potentially useful materials are secretion products including (ectopic) hormones, isoenzymes, oncofoetal antigens and tumour-associated antigens (Chapter 4).

The situation is best understood by considering tumour products which are relatively well analysed and which have real, if limited, value in clinical practice.

Myeloma

The production of Ig molecules or parts of the Ig molecule by myelomas is the best example of this situation. Myeloma is a malignant proliferation of plasma cells and the tumour cells retain their functional differentiation to a degree which is reflected by the nature of their products. Well differentiated tumours produce complete Ig molecules, moderately differentiated tumours fragments of the Ig molecule, and totally dedifferentiated tumours are non-productive. The range of functional differentiation correlates well with tumour behaviour, non-producers being the most malignant tumours. Since the tumour is monoclonal the materials produced are homogeneous and are seen as a defined spike on plasma electrophoresis by comparison with the diffuse general increase of gammaglobulins seen in chronic infections. The abnormal materials are excreted in the urine and may be detected as Bence-Jones protein. The height of the monoclonal electrophoretic spike and its area indicate the amount of abnormal Ig produced and provide a good estimate of the number of myeloma cells present. With the important exception of non-secretory tumours this is thus a simple product based diagnostic technique.

Trophoblastic hormones

Tumours of the trophoblast and teratomas containing trophoblastic elements produce a range of hormones. Techniques such as radioimmunoassay permit their very exact measurement even at low concentration, and the quantities present may be related to the number of tumour cells present. Assays of plasma levels of human chorionic gonadotrophin (HCG) and human placental lactogen (HPL) have proved valuable aids to the diagnosis of gestational trophoblastic tumours and appropriately differentiated teratomas (Bagshawe, 1969). Raised levels of hormone in the cerebrospinal fluid may also be of value in the diagnosis of HCG producing metastases in the central nervous system (Bagshawe and Harland, 1976).

Other hormones

The situation with HCG suggests that the detection of raised levels of other hormones produced by tumours of conventional endocrine organs and "inappropriately" by tumours of non-endocrine organs may be of value in immunodiagnosis.

Oncofoetal (OF) antigens

Carcinoembryonic antigen (CEA) was described by Gold and Freedman in 1965 as a TAA of large bowel cancer, shared with foetal colon cells, but absent from adult colonic cells. On this basis it was considered that raised plasma CEA might be of value in the diagnosis of carcinoma of the colon. Unfortunately subsequent studies with more sensitive techniques have shown CEA at low concentration on adult colonic cells and in normal serum and at raised concentration in the serum of patients with cancer of a variety of sites including the urothelial tract and breast, and of patients with chronic inflammatory bowel disease and chronic liver disease (Laurence *et al.*, 1972). CEA levels were also observed to be raised in well individuals who were heavy cigarette smokers. The demonstration of raised CEA in body fluids is thus insufficiently specific for use in diagnostic screening.

The salutory tale of CEA warns against uncritical or premature attempts to use TAA in cancer diagnosis. This is especially true of oncofoetal antigens and the CEA experience may be repeated with other OF antigens as they are discovered. The situation may be different with true neoantigens induced in tumours by carcinogen contact.

Alpha-fetoprotein (α-FP) is an OF antigen which is raised in the serum of a proportion of patients with primary liver cancer or germ cell tumours (Chapter 4). While some of the problems of specificity encountered with CEA apply to α-FP it has found some application in the assessment of patients suspected of having a hepatoma.

Foetal enzymes which make their (re)appearance in some tumour cells, may also eventually be of some value in tumour diagnosis.

Tumour-associated antigens other than OF antigens (TAA)

Identification and isolation of TAA will permit the production of specific antisera and the development of radioimmunoassays for TAA shed into blood and urine. The applicability of this approach hinges upon the frequency with which human tumours produce antigens which are relatively disease specific: a central and crucial piece of information which remains highly debatable. Since a relatively small number of types of cancer make up the great bulk of malignant disease it might be possible, if TAA are of common occurrence, to prepare a panel of reagents which would react with the cells of a majority of cancers and identify their histogenesis. This would substantially narrow the areas appropriate for detailed scrutiny by radiology and scintigraphy offering a considerable saving of time and expense.

THE INDICES OF TUMOUR-DIRECTED IMMUNE REACTIONS IN DIAGNOSIS

In the absence of tumour markers unique for each tumour and reagents capable of specifically identifying circulating TAA an alternative and currently practical approach to immunodiagnosis is to identify and quantify tumour-directed immunity. Relatively simple techniques exist for this type of study and there are many reports which compare the frequency of reactions in patients with a particular type of cancer and a more or less appropriate control population (Chapter 3). This is theoretically an interesting approach, but its validity depends entirely on the specificity of the reactions detected. A major criticism of many such studies is that the selection of the control populations has been arbitrary and the most appropriate group of individuals, those with non-malignant conditions, the signs and symptoms of which can simulate the relevant cancer and lead to a diagnostic dilemma, has not always been studied.

A further problem is that the tumour antigen source is seldom ideally controlled by the parallel testing of equivalent preparations of the *cell of origin of the tumour* and *in particular* by preparations from the appropriate foetal tissues. Those conducting this type of study are generally aware of these deficiencies but the provision of ideal control material may be impossible. In studies of melanoma the provision of adequate numbers of normal melanocytes as target cells for cytotoxicity or for antigen extraction has proved almost impossible. The one ingenious exception to this was the report by Federman *et al.* (1976) where uveal tract melanocytes were used in a study of anti-melanoma antibodies by immunofluorescence. The provision of foetal melanocytes presents an even more difficult problem. The use of heterogeneous embryonic tissues containing an uncontrolled plethora of antigens is certainly a far from ideal answer to the problem.

Despite the qualifications noted above, it is clear that most adequately conducted studies of tumour directed humoral and cellular immunity in man have shown these indices of reaction to be *relatively* specific for cancer patients. However all are bedevilled by two major problems; reactions which are apparently false-positive or false-negative. A proportion of cancer patients do not react and constitute a false-negative population. There are many possible explanations for this. Patients with advanced disease lose detectable reactivity, however such patients seem unlikely to present a diagnostic problem in practice. Lymphocytes may be affected by blocking factors, or the presence of cytotoxic or other drugs and due allowance must be made for these factors. There appear to be subgroups of TAA and unless patients are tested against a panel of such antigens they may appear non-reactive purely because the antigens employed are inappropriate. Our own experience is that the more preparations we test a melanoma patient against, the more likely is a positive reaction (Figure 6.2A). By contrast the frequency of reactions with melanoma patients or control donors does not increase as the number of control antigens tested is increased (Figure 6.2C and D). The increase in reaction frequency of control leucocytes with increasing number of melanoma preparations is not statistically significant (Figure 6.2B).

Apparently false positive reactions may also be troublesome. Regardless of the technique employed, most studies report 15 to 25% of control individuals as giving a positive reaction. As an example of this, the results of a recent study of tumour-directed cell mediated immunity in breast carcinoma are presented in Table 6.7. Thirty per cent of the 138 breast cancer patients showed no reaction. This was maximum in patients with visceral metastases, 13 of 22 patients in this category (59%) being non-reactive compared with 16 non-reactors in 57 patients with tumour confined to the breast on clinical examination (28%) and 4 non reactors in 31 patients with tumour in the breast and the ipsilateral axillary nodes (12%). Clearly clinical stage is important in determining non-reactivity, however, the existence of almost 30% of non-reactors in the Stage I group points to the existence of other reasons for this. Positive reactions were encountered in only 29 of 157 control donors (19%). The proportion of reactors was similar whether the control donors were individuals with non-malignant breast disease, normal individuals, patients with non tumorous conditions or patients with other cancers.

The most facile explanation is that these reactions are genuinely false, indicating the technical limitations of the methods employed. Another possibility is that the reactions detect lymphocytes which have been activated by, for instance, a virus infection. We have observed apparently tumour-directed reactions (melanoma, breast cancer, neuroblastoma) in normal individuals with an upper respiratory infection. When retested after their virus infection had subsided these individuals gave a consistently negative reaction. Other factors which may affect reactivity include hormone changes associated with menstruation, concurrent medicaments and stress (Chapter 7). An intriguing possibility is that a proportion of the general population are genuinely sensitised to TAA, either by random exposure to carcinogens or by contact with cancer patients. Sensitisation to tumour products has been shown in environment-sharing relatives of patients with neuroblastoma,

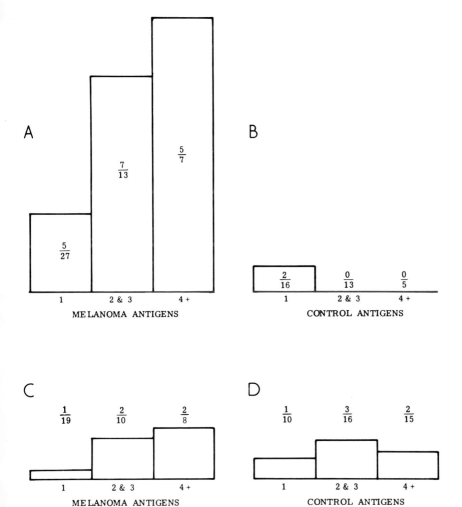

Fig. 6.2. The frequency of reactions of the leucocytes of melanoma patients and control individuals tested against formalinised melanoma cells and formalinised cells from other sources* in a two-stage leucocyte migration assay (Cochran *et al.*, *Pigment Cell*, In Press).
A. melanoma leucocytes   *v*   melanoma cells
B. melanoma leucocytes   *v*   control cells
C. control leucocytes   *v*   melanoma cells
D. control leucocytes   *v*   control cells

———————

*Carcinomas of kidney, ovary and colon; mouse melanoma; normal spleen and normal skin.

Table 6.7.

The incidence of positive and negative reactions in a study of women with breast cancer and control donors by the leucocyte migration technique using breast cancer extracts as "antigen" (Cochran et al., 1974)

Leucocyte donors	Positive reaction[a]		Negative reaction	
	$+/T$[b]	%	$-/T$[c]	%
Breast cancer	97/138	70	41/138	30
Stage I	41/57	72	16/57	28
Stage II	27/31	88	4/27	12
Stage III	9/22	41	13/22	59
Control donors	29/157	19	128/157	81
Simple breast disease	18/96	19	78/96	81
Other control donors	11/61	18	50/61	82

[a]Significant leucocyte migration inhibition and enhancement reactions combined.
[b]Positive reactors over total individuals tested.
[c]Negative reactors over total individuals tested.

osteogenic sarcoma, Burkitt's lymphoma, leukaemia and breast cancer (see Leading Article in Lancet, 1977 for review). Sensitisation has also been shown in close professional contacts of neuroblastoma patients; e.g. paediatric physicians and haematology technicians (Graham-Pole et al., 1976). This situation is reminiscent of that associated with the horizontally transmissible feline leukaemia virus (FeLV) where a proportion of exposed cats get leukaemia and other diseases, including autoimmune disease, but many merely develop antibodies to FeLV and lymphocytes sensitised to FeLV (Hardy et al., 1976).

If control responders are reacting in an immunologically non-specific manner, it is likely that further technological refinements will reduce the frequency of "false-positive" reactions. Such non-specific reactions might be due to the misrecognition of antigens by cells sensitised to antigens other than those on tumour cells, but possessing some degree of structural similarity to them. It is also possible that the false-positive reactions are due to the presence of lymphocytes activated by stimuli other than TAA, such as intercurrent infections and preparative manipulations. If control donors are genuinely sensitised to TAA technological advance will not reduce the size of the group of positive reactors, although it may be possible to detect quantifiable differences in the strength of reaction and number of reactive cells between individuals with tumours and those in the reactive control category.

It would be foolhardy to rely on this type of assay as a sole means of cancer diagnosis but immunodiagnosis will probably become a valuable adjunct to other techniques. We have, for instance, found the combinations of several techniques, the direct (one stage) leucocyte migration assay, a two-stage assay for migration inhibition factor synthesis (lymphocytes plus formalinised tumour cells, supernatant tested on normal leucocytes) and indirect membrane immunofluorescence of tissue cultured melanoma cells a useful addition to conventional diagnostic techniques in patients with detached retina where uveal melanoma is suspected.

It has been considered that the cells comprising the different malignant diseases might share common membrane components which would act as markers for malignancy (as opposed to markers for different kinds of malignancy). Identification of a common cancer antigen, or antibodies or sensitised lymphocytes reactive with it would provide a useful screening technique for detecting cancerous individuals. This is clearly an attractive proposition. However, most such tests have not stood the test of time and with increasing experience initial apparent specificity has dwindled to non-specificity.

It has been claimed (Field and Caspary, 1970) that cancer patients are sensitised to a "cancer basic protein" extractable from a wide variety of tumours and that this reaction may be detected by the macrophage electrophoretic mobility test (Chapter 3). The technology of this approach remains too cumbersome and capricious for routine laboratory use and recent reports have cast doubt upon the cancer specificity of the reactions observed (Lewkonia et al., 1974; Crozier et al., 1976).

An interesting recent development has been the introduction of a commercially produced kit for the diagnosis of cancer.* This employs the technology of the Makari intradermal test (Makari, 1969) in which the intradermal injection of tumour extracted polysaccharides induces an immediate erythematous and oedematous cutaneous response. A considerable degree of specificity has been claimed (Makari and Goddard, 1977) and it will be fascinating to see how the test performs in the hard proving ground of general use.

Monitoring to Detect Recurrences or Metastases Before they Become Clinically Detectable

The early detection of tumour recurrences or metastases would permit the more rational deployment of therapy at a time when the tumour burden is small and maximally vulnerable. Chemotherapy and radiotherapy could be confined to patients with a genuine need for additional treatment and patients without extending disease could be spared the unpleasant side

---

*Ormont Diagnostics Limited, London.

effects of such treatment. However, the provision of effective surveillance remains a major problem in clinical oncology. At present this entails serial clinical examinations, radiology, biochemistry and specialised techniques such as scintigraphy and ultrasonography. The situation remains unsatisfactory as tumour deposits are often not detected until they are beyond the optimum stage for therapy. The requirement is for readily detectable tumour-specific materials which correlate with tumour cell numbers, permitting confidence that fluctuations in level reflect variations in the tumour cell population.

TUMOUR MARKERS

Tumour marker products fulfil some of these criteria and serial assessment of abnormal immunoglobulins in myeloma and of HCG levels in tropho-blastic malignancy are of proven value (Bagshawe and Harland, 1976). CEA has also found a place in the monitoring of patients with carcinoma of the colon (Holyoke et al., 1972; Laurence et al., 1972). A persistently raised plasma CEA after surgical removal of a colon cancer suggests residual tumour and rising levels can be interpreted with some confidence as indicating progressively growing metastases. Urinary levels of CEA may be used in a similar way in cancer of the urothelial tract. (Hall et al., 1972). Alpha-fetoprotein levels have been used with some success in monitoring hepatoma patients (Thompson, 1974). Other potentially useful markers include milk proteins in breast cancer, foetal haemoglobins in leukaemia and calcitonin in medullary carcinoma of the thyroid and it seems likely that many others remain to be discovered and exploited.

SERUM PROTEINS

Other less specific changes in the serum which correlate with tumour presence and growth have been investigated including alpha-globulins (Sarcione, 1967; Ablin, 1972; Suga and Tamura, 1972), haptoglobins (McPhedran, 1972; Douma and Dalen, 1974), alpha[2] H globulin (Rimbaut, 1973) and pregnancy related macroglobulins (Horne et al., 1973; Stimson, 1975). There has also been interest in plasma and urinary polyamines and nucleoside levels (Russell, 1971; Tormey et al., 1975). The lack of tumour specificity of materials of this kind seems likely to cause major problems in interpretation but serial examinations may be of value. It is claimed, for instance, that elevated levels of pregnancy associated macroglobulins can predict breast cancer recurrences by up to twenty one months (Anderson et al., 1976).

INDICES OF TUMOUR-DIRECTED IMMUNE REACTIONS

In the absence of tumour markers it seems reasonable, as in immuno-diagnosis, to consider the utility of serial assessments of anti-tumour immune responses. The number of reports of sequential studies of this kind is increasing rapidly and on balance they suggest that this approach may be practicable (Table 6.8). The many different techniques employed merely reflects the particular enthusiasms of different groups of workers and the absence of pre-eminently excellent techniques. Hellström *et al.* (1973) highlighted the desirability of performing *several tests in parallel in serial studies*. They studied melanoma patients for lymphocytotoxicity, serum cytotoxicity, serum blocking activity and the capacity of serum to "unblock"

Table 6.8.

Some reports of sequential studies of immunological reactions in cancer patients

Techniques	Tumour	Reference
Lymphocytotoxicity	Bladder cancer	O'Toole *et al.* (1972). *Int. J. Cancer* **10**, 77.
Membrane immuno-fluorescence	Burkitt lymphoma	Gunvén *et al.* (1973). *Int. J. Cancer* **12**, 115.
Lymphocytotoxicity, serum cytotoxicity, serum blocking/unblocking	Melanoma	Hellström *et al.* (1972). *Int. J. Cancer* **11**, 280.
Lymphocyte subpopulations (active T cells)	Various	Wybran and Fudenberg (1973). *J. Clin. Invest.* **52**, 1026.
Lymphocyte subpopulations	Bronchial cancer	Anthony *et al.* (1975). *Clin. exp. Immunol.* **20**, 41.
DNCB reactivity	Melanoma and sarcoma	Eilber *et al.* (1975). *Cancer* **35**, 660.
Mitogen transformation lymphocytes	Melanoma	Golub *et al.* (1977). *Int. J. Cancer* **19**, 18.
Leucocyte migration	Breast cancer	Jones and Turnbull (1975). *Br. J. Cancer* **32**, 339.
Lymphocyte subpopulations, mitogen transformation lymphocytes	Carcinoma	Lamelin *et al.* (1977). *Int. J. Cancer* **20**, 723.
Skin tests, recall and tumour antigens	Burkitt lymphoma	Nkrumah *et al.* (1977). *Int. J. Cancer* **20**, 6.
Spontaneous killing of tumour cells by lymphocytes	Melanoma	Saal *et al.* (1977). *Cancer Immunol. Immunother.* **3**, 27.

blocking sera. When tumour was clinically undetectable lymphocytotoxicity and serum cytotoxicity were strong, serum did not block lymphocyte mediated killing and could neutralise other sera with known blocking activity. When tumour was present and growing, lymphocytotoxicity was weak and serum blocked but did not kill target tumour cells.

We currently assess patients monthly by the undernoted tests:—

(a) *The leucocyte migration inhibition test employing formalinised tumour cells as antigen* (Ross *et al.*, 1975)

Initial attempts to correlate this test with clinical events on the basis of a positive or negative reaction (significance assessed by the Mann-Whitney-Wilcoxon U test of ranking) were unsuccessful. Subsequently we plotted the

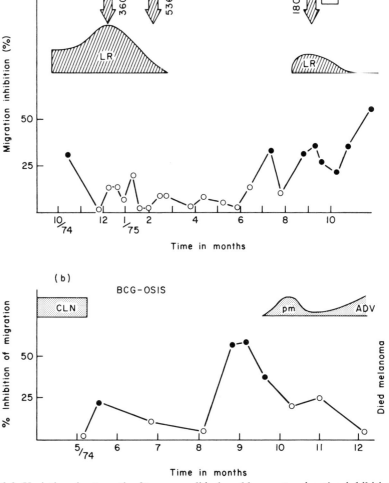

Fig. 6.3. Variations in strength of tumour cell induced leucocyte migration inhibition. (a) Following radiotherapy. LR is locally recurrent tumour. RT is radiotherapy. DTIC is course of imidazole carboxamide. (b) During and following a generalised infection with Bacille Calmette-Guerin. CLN is melanoma in the cervical lymph nodes. PM is tumour in porta hepatis. ADV is progressively advancing systemic metastases.

strength of the reaction (percentage inhibition of migration) and obtained a good clinical correlation. There is a reduction in reaction strength during and following radiotherapy (Fig. 6.3a), during severe intercurrent illness or infective complications of BCG therapy (Fig. 6.3b), transiently following

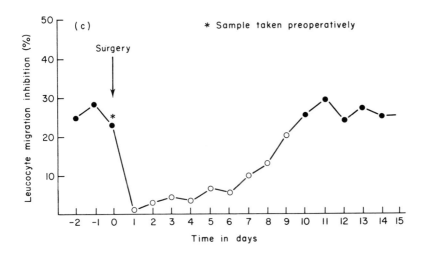

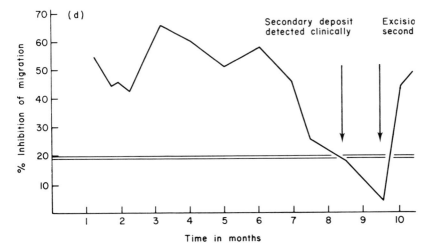

Fig. 6.3 (cont.) (c) Following a surgical operation. (d) Preceding the development of clinically detectable metastatic tumour.
● is statistically significant leucocyte migration inhibition by tumour antigen.
o is non-significant leucocyte migration inhibition by tumour antigen.

surgery (Fig. 6.3c) and most importantly 2 to 6 months prior to the development of metastatic or recurrent disease (Fig. 6.3d).

(b) *A second useful test is to compare leucocyte migration in medium
supplemented with autologous decomplemented serum with that in foetal
calf serum containing medium* (Cochran *et al.*, 1976)

Serum inhibitory activity is absent in patients who are clinically tumour free
but rises transiently prior to (1-4 months) or coincidentally with the
appearance of clinically evident metastases (Fig. 6.4a). Serum inhibitory
activity is also present during periods of tumour breakdown by radiotherapy
and chemotherapy (Fig. 6.4b). The postulated but as yet unproven
mechanism of serum mediated leucocyte migration inhibition is the presence
of antigen-antibody complexes at critical ratio, presumably reflecting
antibody excess as the activity disappears when the volume of tumour
increased. Fractionation of active sera on Sephadex G200 columns suggests
the active materials to have a molecular weight of between 7S and 12S, in
which area immune complexes of 7S antibody would be found.

(c) *The third test is the effect of autologous decomplemented serum (AS) on
leucocyte migration inhibition by formalinised tumour cells* (Cochran *et al.*,
1976)

Three effects are possible. Leucocyte migration inhibition in AS may be
identical to that in foetal calf serum (FCS), greater than in FCS or the
inhibition seen in FCS may be reduced or abolished by AS. The last effect
would seem analogous to the blocking of cellular cytotoxicity described by
others (Chapter 5).

Serum which increased leucocyte migration inhibition induced by
formalinised tumour cells comes most frequently from patients with a small
or medium tumour burden. Sera which block migration inhibition are almost
exclusive to patients with advanced tumour (Table 5.2). The interpretation of
serial studies of this type of serum effect is difficult as the values are derived
from two variables; leucocyte inhibition by FTC and the activity of AS and at
present we rely more on the variations in tests (a) and (b) to predict
metastases. At the time of writing this approach has accurately predicted
metastases in 22 of 24 patients (Unpublished data).

While the techniques at present available are cumbersome I am confident
that this type of approach, employing simpler technology, will find a place in
the management of cancer patients in the relatively near future. Immunological monitoring is clearly in its infancy, is extremely time consuming and
interpretation of results requires very careful consideration of the effects of a
growing or regressing tumour, which may of itself be immunosuppressive, the
effects of specific anti-tumour therapy, and the effect of concurrent medical

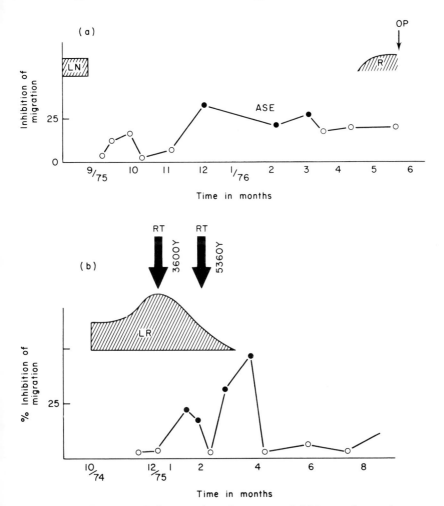

Fig. 6.4. Development of the capacity of serum to inhibit autologous leucocyte migration (in the absence of added tumour antigen). (a) Prior to the development of clinically detectable metastases. LN is lymph node recurrence. R. is further nodal metastases. ASE is autologous serum effect. (b) After tumour reduction by radiotherapy. Lr is locally recurrent melanoma. RT is radiotherapy.
● is statistically significant leucocyte migration inhibition by autologous serum.
o is statistically non-significant leucocyte migration inhibition by autologous serum.

conditions either independent of or consequent upon the tumour or its treatment. The value of a system of monitoring which could predict recurrent disease before it became clinically apparent, provides adequate justification for the continued examination of immunological phenomena in cancer

Table 6.9.

Some reports indicating that the prognosis of cancer patients correlates with immunological competence

Tests	Cancer	Reference
Response to BCG vaccination	Hodgkin's disease	Sokal and Aungst (1969). *Cancer* **24**, 128.
DNCB sensitisation	Melanoma	Morton *et al.* (1970). *Surgery* **68**, 159.
Skin reaction to tumour antigen	Burkitt lymphoma	Bluming *et al.* (1971),
Lymphocyte count	Hodgkin's disease	Swan and Knowelden (1971). *Brit. J. Haematol.* **21**, 343.
DNCB sensitisation	Colon carcinoma	Bone and Camplejohn (1973). *Brit. J. Surg.* **60**, 824.
DNCB sensitisation	Various cancers	Chakravorty *et al.* (1973). *Surgery* **73**, 730.
PHA blastogenesis	Various carcinomas	Chretien *et al.* (1973). *Surg. Gynec. Obstet.* **136**, 380.
DNCB sensitisation PHA blastogenesis	Breast cancer	Hoge *et al.* (1973). *Amer. J. Surg.* **126**, 722.
Tuberculin positivity	Lung cancer	Israel *et al.* (1973). *Biomed.* **19**, 68.
Reduced 'active' T lymphocytes	Melanoma	Wybran and Spitler (1973). *Clin. Res.* **21**, 655.
Recall skin tests PHA blastogenesis	Hodgkin's disease	Young *et al.* (1973). *Arch. intern. Med.* **131**, 446.
Recall skin tests	Various carcinomas	Romieu and Serrou (1974). *Bull. Acad. Nat. de Med.* **158**, 71.
Reduced "active" T lymphocytes	Melanoma	Claudy *et al.* (1975). *Europ. J. Cancer*
Lymphocytotoxicity	Bladder cancer	Elhilali and Nayak (1975). *Cancer* **35**, 419.
Recall skin tests DNCB sensitisation Blastogenesis and MLC[a]	Lung cancer	Holmes and Golub (1976). *J. Thorac. Cardiovasc. Surg.* **71**, 161.
Leucocyte migration inhibition	Prostatic cancer	Ablin *et al.* (1977). *IRCS Med. Sci.* **5**, 57.

[a]MLC = mixed lymphocyte culture reaction.

patients, even if, from a biological standpoint, such phenomena are merely epiphenomena and have no significant or major inhibitory activity against spontaneous tumours *in vivo*.

The Relationship Between Immunological Competence, Anti-Tumour Immunity and Prognosis

The great majority of authors who report on studies relating the results of immunological assessment to prognosis have found a positive correlation between immunological competence and favourable prognosis (Table 6.9). This is true whether the study assessed general parameters of immunological function, immunological memory, the capacity to mount a new immune response or anti-tumour immunity. There is thus a strong argument in favour of the immunological assessment of cancer patients *before the initiation of treatment*. However the improvement in prognosis is only relative and this type of evaluation must be interpreted in relation to other significant prognostic factors, especially the extent of tumour spread assessed by clinical examination, radiology and scintigraphy.

It would be very desirable to know the extent to which immunological competence predicts response to or tolerance of therapy. Little is known of this important relationship and it is certainly an area where concentrated research effort is desirable and likely to yield information of practical value. This subject is discussed in Chapter 7.

References

Ablin, R. J. (1972). *Lancet* **2**, 874.

Ablin, R. J., Gordon, M. J. and Soane, W. A. (1972). *Neoplasma* **19**, 57-60.

Allison, A. C. (1972). *Ann. Inst. Pasteur* **123**, 585.

Amos, D. B., Hattler, B. G. and Shingleton, W. W. (1965). *Lancet* **1**, 414-415.

Anderson, J. M., Stimson, W. H. and Kelly, F. (1976). *Brit. J. Surg.* **63**, 819.

Ashburn, P., Cooper, M. R., McCall, C. E. and De Chatelet, L. R. (1973). *Blood* **41**, 921.

Baehner, R. L., Neiburger, R. G., Johnson, D. E. and Murrman, S. M. (1973). *New Engl. J. Med.* **289**, 1209.

Bagshawe, K. D. (1969). "Choriocarcinoma: the Clinical Biology of the Trophoblast and its Tumours." Edward Arnold, London.

Bagshawe, K. D. and Harland, S. (1976). *Cancer* **38**, 112.

Bandilla, K. K., McDuffie, F. C. and Gleich, G. J. (1969). *Clin. exp. Immunol.* **5**, 627.

Barkas, T., Al-Khateeb, S. F., Irvine, W. J., Davidson, N. M. and Roscoe, P. (1976). *Clin. exp. Immunol.* **25**, 270.

Baude, A. I., Feltes, J. and Brooks, M. (1954). *J. Clin. Invest.* **33**, 1036.

Bernier, G. M. (1964). *Amer. J. Med.* **36**, 618.

Catalona, W. J., Sample, W. F. and Chretien, P. B. (1973). *Cancer* **31**, 65.

Chakravorty, R. C., Curutcher, H. P., Coppolla, F. S., Choon, M. P., Blaycock, W. K. and Lawrence, W. (1973). *Surg.* **73**, 730.

Chang, S. (1967). *Jap. J. exp. Med.* **37**, 97.

Claudy, A. L., Viac, J., Pelletier, N., Fouad-Wassef, N., Alario, A. and Thivolet, J. (1976). *In* "Clinical Tumour Immunology" (J. Wybran and M. J. Staquet, Eds.). Pergamon Press, Oxford.

Cline, M. J. (1973). *J. Lab. Clin. Med.* **81**, 311.

Cochran, A. J., Mackie, R. M., Ross, C. E., Ogg, L. J. and Jackson, A. M. (1976). *Int. J. Cancer* **18**, 274.

Cochran, A. J., Mackie, R. M., Grant, R. M., Ross, C. E., Connell, M. D., Sandilands, G., Whaley, K., Hoyle, D. E. and Jackson, A. M. (1976). *Int. J. Cancer* **18**, 298.

Crowther, D., Hamilton Fairley, G. and Sewell, R. L. (1969). *Brit. med. J.* **2,** 473.
Crozier, E. H., Hollinger, M. E., Woodend, B. E. and Robertson, J. H. (1976). *J. Clin. Path.* **29,** 608.
deGast, G. C. (1975). "Immune responsiveness in patients with malignant melanoma." Thesis of The University of Groningen.
Dellon, A. L., Potoin, C. and Chretien, P. B. (1975). *Cancer* **35,** 687.
Donma, G. J. and Dalen, van A. (1974). *Zeit. Klin. Chem. Klin. Biochim.* **12,** 474.
Eilber, F. R. and Morton, D. L. (1970). *Cancer* **25,** 362.
Epstein, W. L. and Kligmann, A. M. (1959). *J. invest. Derm.* **33,** 231.
Evans, R. and Alexander, P. (1972). *Immunology* **23,** 615.
Fahey, J. L. (1965). *J. Amer. Med. Ass.* **194,** 255-258.
Fakhri, O., McLaughlin, H. and Hobbs, J. R. (1973). *Europ. J. Cancer* **9,** 19.
Federman, J. L., Lewis, M. G. and Clark, W. H. (1974). *J. nat. Cancer Inst.* **52,** 587.
Feldman, M. (1969). *J. exp. Med.* **135,** 1049.
Field, E. J. and Caspary, E. A. (1970). *Lancet* **2,** 1337.
Gold, P., Freedman, S. O. (1965). *J. exp. Med.* **121,** 439-462.
Golub, S. H., O'Connell, T. X. and Morton, D. L. (1974). *Cancer Res.* **34,** 1833-1837.
Graham-Pole, J., Ogg, L. J., Ross, C. E. and Cochran, A. J. (1976). *Lancet* **1,** 1376-1379.
Groch, G. S., Perillie, P. E. and Finch, S. C. (1965). *Blood* **26,** 489.
Gross, R. L., Latty, A., Williams, E. A. and Newberne, P. M. (1975). *New Engl. J. Med.* **292,** 439.
Hall, R. R., Laurence, D. J. R., Cardy, D., Stevens, U., James, R., Roberts, S. and Neville, A. M. (1972). *Brit. med. J.* **3,** 609-611.
Hamilton, D. N. H., Ledger, V. and Diamandopoulos, A. (1976). *Lancet* **4,** 1170-1171.
Han, T. and Takita, H. (1972). *New Engl. J. Med.* **186,** 605-606.
Hardy, W. D., Hess, P. W., MacEwen, G., McLelland, A. J., Zuckerman, E. E., Essex, M., Cotter, S. M. and Jarrett, O. (1976). *Cancer Res.* **36,** 582.
Hellström, I., Warner, G. A., Hellström, K. E. and Sjögren, H. O. (1973). *Int. J. Cancer* **11,** 280-292.
Hersh, E. M. and Oppenheim, J. (1965). *New Engl. J. Med.* **273,** 1006-1012.
Holyoke, D., Reynoso, G. and Chu, T. M. (1972). *Ann. Surg.* **176,** 559-564.
Horne, C. H. W., McLay, A. L. C., Tavadia, H. B., Carmichael, I., Mallinson, A. C., Yeung Laiwah, A. A. C., Thomas, M. A. and MacSween, R. N. M. (1973). *Clin. Exper. Immunol.* **13,** 603.
Hughes, I. E. and McKay, W. D. (1965). *Brit. med. J.* **1,** 1346-1348.
Humphrey, G. B., Peterson, L., Whalen, M., Parker, D. E., Lankford, J., Krivit, W. (1975). *Cancer* **35,** 1341.
Inai, S., Fuyikawa, K. and Magakik *et al.* (1967). *Biken J.* **10,** 65.
Jewell, D. P. and McLennan, I. C. M. (1973). *Clin. exp. Immunol.* **14,** 219.
Karlinske, R. W. and Hoeprich, P. D. (1969). *Cancer* **23,** 1094.
Kent, J. F. and Fife, E. H. (1963). *Amer. J. Trop. Med. Hyg.* **12,** 103.
Keusch, G., Douglas, S. D. and Mildvan, D. (1972). *Infect. Immun.* **5,** 414.
Knight, L. A. and Davidson, W. M. (1975). *J. Clin. Path.* **28,** 372.
Kopersztych, S., Rezkallah, M. T., Naspitz, C. K. and Mendes, N. F. (1976). *Cancer* **38,** 1149-1154.
Krant, M. J., Manskopf, G., Brandrup, C. S. and Madoff, M. A. (1968). *Cancer* **21,** 623.
Lamb, D., Pilney, F., Kelley, W. D. and Good, R. A. (1962). *J. Immunol.* **89,** 555.

Laurence, D. J. R., Stevens, U., Bettelheim, R., Darcy, D., Leese, C., Turberville, C., Alexander, P., Johns, E. W. and Neville, A. M. (1972). *Brit. med. J.* **3**, 605-609.

Laurel, C. B. (1965). *Analyt. Biochem.* **10**, 358.

Leading Article (1977). *Lancet* **1**, 635.

Lee, J. C., Yamauchi, H. and Hopper, J. (1966). *Ann. int. Med.* **64**, 41.

Lejeune, F. J. (1975). *Biomedicine* **22**, 25.

Levin, A. G., McDonough, E. G., Miller, D. G. and Southam, C. M. (1964). *Ann. N.Y. Acad. Sci.* **120**, 400.

Lewkonia, R. M., Kerr, L. and Irvine, W. J. (1974). *Brit. J. Cancer* **30**, 532-537.

Lonai, P. and Feldman, M. (1971). *Immunology* **21**, 861.

Loughbridge, L. and Lewis, M. G. (1971). *Lancet* **1**, 256.

Lytton, B., Hughes, L. E. and Fulthorpe, A. J. (1964). *Lancet* **1**, 69-71.

Mackie, R. M., Cochran, A. J., Ogg, L. J., Jackson, A. M., Ross, C. E. and Todd, G. (1977). *Pigment Cell.* (In Press.)

Makari, J. G. (1969). *J. Am. Geriatric Soc.* **17**, 755-789.

Makari, J. G. and Goddard, J. L. (1977) "Proceedings of the 3rd International Symposium on Detection and Prevention of Cancer." Marcel Dekler, New York.

Mancini, G., Carbonara, A. O. and Heremans, J. F. (1965). *Immunochem.* **2**, 235.

Mandel, M. A., Dvorak, K. and deCosse, J. (1973). *Cancer* **31**, 1408-1413.

Mayer, M. M. (1961). *In* "Experimental Immunochemistry, 2nd Edition, pp 133-240 (Kabat, E. A. and Mayer, M. M., Eds.). Thomas, Springfield.

Meier, E. L. and Grob, P. J. (1972). *Dtsch. Med. Wchschr.* **97**, 967.

Miller, D. R. and Kaplan, H. G. (1970). *Pediatrics* **45**, 861.

Miller, A. E. and Levis, W. R. (1973). *J. invest. Derm.* **61**, 261.

McIvor, K. L. and Weiser, R. S. (1971). *Immunology* **20**, 315.

McKenzie, D., Colsky, J. and Hetrick, L. (1967). *Cancer Res.* **27**, 2386.

McPhedran, P. (1972). *Ann. int. Med.* **76**, 439.

Nelson, H. S. (1969). *J. nat. Cancer Inst.* **42**, 765-770.

Nemoto, T., Han, T., Minowada, J. *et al.* (1974). *J. nat. Cancer Inst.* **53**, 641-645.

Otu, A. A., Russell, R. J., Wilkinson, P. C. and White, R. G. (1977). *Brit. J. Cancer* **36**, 330.

Park, B. H., Fikrig, S. M. and Smithwick, E. M. (1968). *Lancet* **2**, 532.

Paty, D. W. and Bone, G. (1973). *Lancet* **1**, 668-669.

Pickering, L. K., Anderson, D. C., Sung, C. and Feigin, R. D. (1975). *Cancer* **35**, 1365.

Plager, J. and Stutzman, L. (1971). *Amer. J. Med.* **50**, 56.

Plesnicar, S. (1972). *Acta Radiol.* **11**, 34-47.

Rimbaut, C. (1973). *Bull. du Cancer* **60**, 411.

Roberts, M. M. (1970). *Brit. J. Surg.* **57**, 381.

Roberts, M. M., Bass, E. M., Wallace, I. W. *et al.* (1973). *Brit. J. Cancer* **27**, 269-275.

Roitt, I. M., Greaves, M. F., Torrigiani, G., Brostoff, J. and Playfair, J. H. L. (1969). *Lancet* **2**, 367.

Rosato, L. O. J. F. E., Brow, A. S., Miller, E. E., Rosato, E. F., Mulus, W. F. and Johnson, S. (1974). *Surg. Gynec. Obstet.* **139**, 675-682.

(1974). *Surg. Gynec. Obstet.* **139**, 675-682.

Rosner, F., Valmont, I., Kozinn, D. J. and Caroline, L. (1970). *Cancer* **25**, 835.

Ross, C. E., Cochran, A. J., Hoyle, D. E., Grant, R. M. and Mackie, R. M. (1975). *Clin. exp. Immunol.* **22**, 126.

Russell, D. H. (1971). *Nature (New Biol.)* **233**, 144-145.
Sample, W. F., Gertner, H. R. and Chretien, P. B. (1971). *J. nat. Cancer Inst.* **46**, 1291.
Sandilands, G. P., Gray, K., Cooney, A., Browning, J. D. and Anderson, J. R. (1975). *Clin. exp. Immunol.* **22**, 493.
Sarcione, E. J. (1967). *Cancer Res.* **27**, 2025.
Silver, R. T., Beal, G. A., Schneiderman, M. A. and McCullough, N. B. (1957). *Blood* **12**, 814.
Skeel, R. T., Yankee, R. A. and Henderson, E. S. (1971). *J. Lab. Clin. Med.* **77**, 975.
Smith, R. T. (1972). *New Engl. J. Med.* **287**, 439-450.
Snyderman, R., Pike, M. C., Blaylock, B. L. and Weinstein, P. (1976). *J. Immunol.* **116**, 585.
Sobel, A. T., Bokisch, V. A. and Muller-Eberhard, H. J. (1975). *J. exp. Med.* **142**, 139.
Solowey, A. C. and Rapaport, F. T. (1965). *Surg. Gynec. Obstet.* **121**, 756-762.
Southam, C. M. and Goldsmith, Y. (1951). *Proc. Soc. Exp. Biol. Med.* **76**, 430.
Southam, C. M. and Siegel, A. H. (1966). *J. Immunol.* **97**, 331.
Stein, J. A., Adler, A., Efraim, S. B. and Maor, M. (1976). *Cancer* **38**, 1171-1187.
Stimson, W. H. (1975). *J. Clin. Path.* **28**, 868-871.
Strauss, R. R., Paul, B. B., Jacobs, A. A., Simmons, C. and Sbarra, A. J. (1970). *Cancer Res.* **30**, 480.
Sucia-Foca, N., Buda, J., McManus, J., Thiem, T. and Reemtsma, K. (1973). *Cancer Res.* **33**, 2373-2377.
Suga, S. and Tamura, Z. (1972). *Cancer Res.* **32**, 426.
Swanson, M. A. and Schwartz, R. S. (1967). *New Engl. J. Med.* **277**, 163.
Tan, C. V., Rosner, F. and Feldman, F. (1973). *N. Y. State J. Med.* **73**, 952.
Thompson, R. A. and Lachmann, P. J. (1970). *J. exp. Med.* **131**, 629.
Thompson, W. G. (1974). *Canad. med. Ass. J.* **110**, 775.
Tormey, D. C., Waalkes, T. P., Ahmann, D., Gehrke, C. W., Zumwatt, R. W., Snyder, J. and Hansen, H. (1975). *Cancer* **35**, 1095-1100.
Uhr, J. W., Dancis, J., Franklin, E. C., Finkelstein, M. S. and Lewis, E. W. (1962). *J. Clin. Invest.* **41**, 509.
Verhaegen, H., deCock, W., de Cree, J. and Verbruggen, F. (1976). *Cancer* **38**, 1608-1613.
Waldmann, A., Strober, W. and Blaese, M. (1972). *Ann. intern. Med.* **77**, 605-628.
Wara, W. M., Wara, D. W., Phillips, T. L. and Ammann, A. J. (1975). *Cancer* **35**, 1313-1315.
Wells, S. A. Jr., Melewicz, F. C., Christiansen, C. *et al.* (1973). *Surg. Gynec. Obstet.* **136**, 717-720.
Whittaker, M. G., Rees, K. and Clark, C. G. (1971). *Lancet* **1**, 892.
Wilkins, S. A. and Olkowski, Z. L. (1977). *Cancer* **39**, 487-488.
Wybran, J. and Fudenberg, H. H. (1973). *J. Clin. Invest.* **52**, 1026.
Yoshida, T. O. and Ito, Y. (1968). *Immunology* **14**, 879.

7

The Effects of Treatment
on the Immune System

There are two main questions to be answered. First, is there any evidence that conventional forms of cancer therapy increase or diminish the activity of the immune system, to an extent which is reflected by events at the clinical level such as increased or slowed tumour progression or increased susceptibility to infection? Second, can we identify techniques which will induce an increase in general and (tumour) specific immunity and if so are such manipulations associated with an improved prognosis? The present chapter will discuss information which relates to the first question. The second question is the subject of Chapter 8.

Management of cancer patients is currently based upon the long established techniques of surgery and radiation therapy and the newer approaches of chemotherapy. The patient may, however, receive other drugs for cancer related problems and intercurrent conditions and it is the overall effect of this polypharmacy and the interaction of its various components on immunity which must be assessed. The situation may be further compounded by nutritional problems leading to deficiency of minerals, vitamins or calories.

Codes of practice for these forms of therapy derive from a vast experience of cancer patients and there is no doubt that their skilful employment offers the best hope of cancer cure presently available. The comments which follow should not be interpreted as an attempt to diminish the value of the established methods of cancer treatment. Clinicians are well aware that these treatments are associated with undesirable morbidity and mortality. As with all forms of medical management, the decision to treat is a compromise between the likelihood of a favourable result, the possibility of morbidity and the risk of death.

In the past considerations of therapy induced morbidity have concentrated on the mechanical and infective complications of surgical operations, the effects of marrow depression induced by radiation or chemotherapy and damage to other organs by these agencies, and the possibility that long term survivors of radiation or chemotherapy might later develop a second, iatrogenic malignancy. There has recently been increasing attention to the effects of therapy on the immunological apparatus. It can readily be shown that standard therapies alter the results of *in vitro* tests of immunological activity and may modify lymphocyte and macrophage numbers, distribution and functional activity. We are, however, remarkably ignorant of the extent to which these alterations, mainly detected *in vitro*, affect local tumour progression and metastasis formation and render the patient susceptible to intercurrent disease. The patient who receives immunosuppressive therapy is certainly at increased risk of infection and the proportion of treated leukaemic patients who succumb to infections with microorganisms which are not lethal to the immunologically intact individual must be regarded as representing the extreme effects of therapy induced immune suppression. Relatively little is known of the effect of therapy induced immune suppression on tumour progression in man. It is possible that in a (probably large) proportion of patients altered immunological parameters are not of sinister significance, perhaps because of the considerable reserve capacity of the immune system and the existence of alternative pathways. Reports of therapy linked enhanced tumour growth are few but the protean behaviour of human cancer means that enhancement could only be identified in controlled clinical trials. The possibility that even a few patients are damaged by standard treatment is a clear indication for urgent investigations to determine whether therapy linked immune suppression can be the cause of this disaster. We need to know the relative effect of different sources and dosages of radiant energy and of different doses, frequencies, combinations and routes of administration of chemotherapy. We also lack information on the cell populations affected by different therapies and the exact duration of the effects they induce. The clinical significance of different degrees, durations and patterns of immune suppression requires to be investigated and the boundaries of acceptable immunological depression should be identified. Techniques may require modifications of timing, dose and extent to maintain immune suppression within acceptable limits and new agents and techniques may need to be developed to counteract situations where severe immune suppression is the unavoidable concomitant of necessary anti-cancer therapy.

Studies of these problems have only recently been initiated and the scale and scope of the questions to be answered makes it unlikely that answers will be rapidly attainable. Nonetheless the nature of the problem dictates urgency in the prosecution of such investigations.

Paucity of information makes this a short chapter but equivalent sections in future books of this kind will certainly be markedly longer.

The Effects of Surgery

Surgical operations induce complex alterations in the patients' physiology and biochemistry, alterations akin to those associated with severe trauma (Howard and Simmons, 1974; Munster and Artz, 1974). That the immunological system is also affected is indicated by reports of transient post-operative depression of (T) lymphocyte transformation by PHA (Riddle and Berenbaum, 1967; Park et al., 1971; Han, 1972) and PPD (Berenbaum et al., 1973) and reduced leucocyte migration inhibition by PPD (Bancewicz et al., 1973).

In a recent study of post surgical immunodepression we investigated 13 breast cancer patients and 12 melanoma patients serially over the operative period by the leucocyte migration inhibition assay for evidence of a decline of *tumour directed* cell-mediated immunity (Cochran et al., 1972). We found that patients who reacted positively preoperatively were non-reactive for a period of 3 to 22 days following the operation, after which reactivity returned to preoperative levels (Table 7.1). This finding has since been confirmed by McCoy et al. (1975) using the leucocyte migration inhibition assay and by Vose and Moudgil (1975, 1976) using lymphocytotoxicity and antibody dependent cell-mediated cytotoxicity assays. All studies to the present suggest that the reduction of tumour directed immunity is merely part of a general post operative immune depression which varies with the degree of operative trauma (Berenbaum et al., 1973; Munster, 1976). The effect appears to be cumulative and a patient who has three surgical operations on

Table 7.1.

Post-operative loss and recovery of tumour antigen induced leucocyte migration inhibition

Tumour type	Post-operative abolition M.I.[a]	Subsequent recovery M.I.[a]	Time to return of M.I. (days)	
			Mean	Range
Melanoma	12/12	11/12	11	6-22
Breast cancer	13/13	7/7	7	3-10
All	25/25	18/19	10	3-22

[a]M.I. is leucocyte migration inhibition by tumour antigen.

three successive weeks, for instance a biopsy, followed by a radical excision, followed by skin grafting, will remain immunologically non-reactive for a total of 28-40 days.

Studies of the mechanisms of this effect have thus far been inconclusive. The intra-operative release of steroids from the adrenal cortex, agents known to have immunosuppressive properties has been considered as a potentially important factor. The kinetics of corticosteroid release and depressed (tumour-specific) immunity are however quite different and it thus appears that if steroids are involved they must induce relatively long lasting effects on the lymphocytes, effects which persist beyond the period of raised circulating steroid levels (Fig. 7.1) (Mackie *et al.*, 1972; Munster *et al.*, 1972; Leguit *et al.*, 1973). Further evidence against a major role for steroids is provided by the observation that post traumatic immune depression may be observed in adrenalectomised animals (Munster *et al.*, 1972).

Anaesthetic agents can depress lymphocyte function *in vitro* (Wingard *et al.*, 1967; Humphrey *et al.*, 1970; Nunn *et al.*, 1970; Bruce and Wingard, 1971; Espanol *et al.*, 1974). The significance of this effect *in vivo* remains very doubtful. In our own study of post-operative immune depression we could not relate the observed immune depression to particular anaesthetic agents or to their routes or duration of administration. In animal studies Cooper *et al.* (1974) found the effect of anaesthesia (Pentobarbitone) to be minimal and Viljanen *et al.* (1973) found anaesthetics to have no effect on primary and secondary immune responses in chickens.

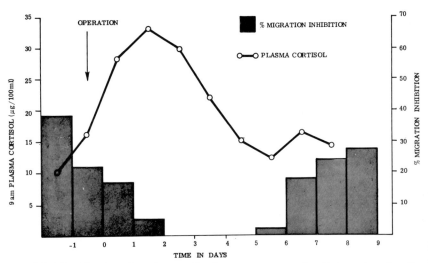

Fig. 7.1. The kinetics of post operative immune suppression (leucocyte migration assay) and alterations of circulating control levels during and after surgery (Mackie *et al.*, 1972).

The production of immunosuppressive materials in damaged tissues is also a possibility and substances of this kind have been extracted from traumatised tissues (Schoenenberger *et al.*, 1975) and identified in the serum of trauma patients (Constantian *et al.*, 1975). There is general agreement that T cells are more affected than B cells and Cooper *et al.* (1974) suggest that it is those stages of the immune response which require T cells to cooperate with other cells that are most affected. Munster (1976) suggests that the immune depression is due to activation of T-suppressor cells and postulates this to be a means of minimising autoimmune reactions to antigens exposed after injury.

The clinical significance of these observations is unknown. It is of interest that tumour directed cell-mediated immunity, including effector cells with the capacity to kill tumour cells *in vitro* is eclipsed at a time when small numbers of tumour cells may have been dislodged and disseminated by operative manipulations. It is certainly possible that this "window" in the host defence may permit tumour cells to establish themselves in areas remote from the operation site, and such escaped cells may be the basis of latent metastases. Most surgeons can recall an occasional patient who rapidly developed disseminated metastases after surgery for an ostensibly localised cancer, and in such (fortunately rare) cases operation-related immune depression may be important. It is perhaps relevant that rats show an increased acceptance of tumour grafts after a surgical operation (Buinauskas *et al.*, 1965).

The Effects of Radiation Therapy

Radiation therapy depresses lymphocyte numbers and some lymphocyte activities to a considerable extent and for very extended periods of time. That these alterations are associated with clinically significant immune deficiency in most patients is far from certain. Opportunistic infection, an excellent marker of significantly reduced host defences, is certainly less common in patients treated with radiotherapy than in those treated by chemotherapy.

There is rare unanimity in the finding that the lymphocyte count is depressed after radiation (Goswitz *et al.*, 1963; Buckston *et al.*, 1967; Stjernswärd *et al.*, 1972; Blomgren *et al.*, 1974 and many others). Lymphopenia may be detected after doses of radiation as low as 25 rads whole body irradiation (Suter, 1947) and is prolonged, reduced levels being detectable five years or more after radiation in patients cured of seminomas (Heier *et al.*, 1975).

In the light of modern thinking on the nature and function of lymphocyte subpopulations it is desirable to know which populations are most affected by radiation. A number of studies of this problem have been undertaken, but have unfortunately resulted in a distinctly confused situation. Initial reports (Stjernswärd et al., 1972; Humphrey et al., 1972; Campbell et al., 1973) found the reduction to be predominantly of T lymphocytes. This finding is to some extent supported by a reduced capacity of the lymphocytes of irradiated individuals to respond to the (predominantly) T mitogen phytohaemagglutinin (Millard, 1965; Ilbery et al., 1971; Thomas et al., 1971; Chee et al., 1974; Dubois et al., 1975). Reduced PHA responsiveness was not, however, a universal finding in other studies (McCredie et al., 1972; Blomgren et al., 1974a and b) which suggested that the lymphopenia after radiation was not exclusively due to T cell reduction. Blomgren et al. (1976) using rosetting techniques and mitogen transformations examined a situation identical to that in which Stjernswärd et al (1972) had found T cell depression and reported the opposite—predominant B cell depression. The same authors also found post irradiation B lymphocyte depression in a study of bladder and prostatic cancer (Blomgren et al., 1974b). Post irradiation B cell reduction has also been recorded in seminoma (Heier et al., 1975) and Hodgkin's disease (Engesett et al., 1973). These paradoxical findings are disquieting but reflect the unsatisfactorily complex techniques presently employed in assessing lymphocyte subpopulations. Specifically it has been suggested that the difference between the findings of Stjernswärd and Blomgren lies in the fact that Blomgren removed monocytes from the mononuclear cell populations studied and Stjernswärd did not. It is claimed that absence of this purification step would lead to an artificially high count of cells reacting like B lymphocytes. That other classes of lymphocytes are affected is shown by the reduced K cell activity recorded by Campbell et al. (1973).

The effects of radiation on skin test reactivity, against primary and recall antigens, are comparatively minor unless one compares reactivity in the skin of an irradiated area with that in skin which has not received radiation (Stjernswärd, 1972). Check et al. (1973) found reduced skin reactivity to mumps antigen after radiation but as this was more pronounced in patients with Hodgkin's disease than in those with carcinoma of the cervix, characteristics of the presenting disease may well be important. Others found little alteration of reaction to DNCB (Gross et al., 1973) or recall antigens (Clements and Kramer, 1974) after radiotherapy and Ghossein et al. (1975) found more patients to convert from DNCB negativity to positivity than the reverse after radiation.

We have found leucocyte migration inhibition by tumour associated antigens to be abolished or severely weakened after radiotherapy and this reduction may persist for many months (Figure 6.3a).

Changes in circulating Ig and in complement levels after radiation have generally been slight (Sohl and Ghossein, 1971; Vasudevan et al., 1971;

Brown *et al.*, 1975; Meyer *et al.*, 1973) but Einhorn *et al.* (1972) found an increase in titre of antibodies to antigens associated with Epstein Barr virus in the months following radiotherapy administered to patients with Burkitt lymphoma, nasopharyngeal carcinoma and maxillary carcinoma. This may represent enhanced immunisation by antigens released during radiation-induced tumour breakdown.

The mechanism of immune depression seems to be predominantly a direct effect of radiant energy on lymphocytes in tissues and circulating through the blood vessels of the irradiated field. If a significant part of the effect is due to damage to transitting lymphocytes, it may be possible to reduce the damage to these cells by using fractionated high doses during a short period. Immunosuppressive materials released from damaged tissues may also be involved. It has been suggested that irradiation of the thymus is associated with the induction of sustained lymphopenia, but recent reports are against this (Stratton *et al.*, 1975; Slater *et al.*, 1976). Irradiation of the bone marrow, on the other hand, is associated with prolonged lymphopenia (Rubin *et al.*, 1973) probably as a result of depletion of lymphocyte reserves.

The evidence that the immunological alterations outlined above produce major immunoincompetence *in vivo* is very slim. Opportunistic infection, as noted previously, is relatively uncommon in irradiated patients and infection is not a specially common cause of death in such patients. Evidence of any deleterious effects of radiotherapy (and other forms of treatment) will not be obtained from studies of the immunology of cancer patients. It is more likely that any such observation will emerge from the analysis of controlled clinical trials and radiotherapists are doubtless well aware of the need to identify the negative as well as the positive results of their endeavours. There is at present no overwhelming evidence that radiotherapy decreases survival in cancer patients so treated, whether as a result of immune depression or any other mechanisms. Stjernswärd *et al.* (1972) amalgamated the results of several separate studies and claimed that radiotherapy does not improve the long term survival of women with breast carcinoma and may increase the likelihood of metastases within the first year after therapy. If this contention is correct and in the light of evidence of depressed immunological function after radiotherapy, it is possible that poor prognosis and immune depression may be linked. Possible as this association may be, much further data is required to substantiate it fully. Since the spectre has been raised, it must be laid, and this will best be done by relating carefully collated survival figures from controlled clinical trials of radiotherapy to results from *in vitro* and *in vivo* studies of general and tumour directed immunity. Alexander (1976) in a plea against "therapeutic nihilism" advocates that "hypothetical considerations of immunity do not justify under-treatment" but in the same paper argues that "all reasonable steps should be taken to maintain the cancer patients' immune capacity at as high a level as possible".

While the clinical significance of post radiation alterations of immuno-logical activity remains unproven there is little doubt that irradiated tissues have a reduced capacity to resist infection, indicated by the development of herpes zoster in irradiated patients with Hodgkin's disease (Sokal and Firat, 1965). Such tissues also show a susceptibility to tumour growth as for example where breast carcinoma recurrences selectively colonise areas of irradiated skin (Fig. 7.2). Whether this increased susceptibility to infection and tumour growth has a purely immunological basis remains to be ascertained.

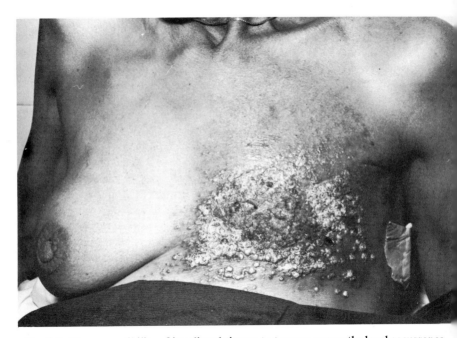

Fig. 7.2. The susceptibility of irradiated tissues to tumour regrowth; local recurrence of breast cancer predominantly confined to an area which had received therapeutic irradiation.

Radiant energy has long been known to be capable of causing cancer. In man it has been incriminated in the aetiology of skin cancers (Hall, 1973), thyroid cancer (Hempelmann, 1968) and leukaemia (Court Brown and Doll, 1957). While direct mutagenesis is undoubtedly the main mechanism of carcinogenesis it is of interest to speculate whether immune suppression may have some relevance.

As a final and relatively optimistic comment on the subject of radiation and immunity it is noteworthy that there is current interest in the prevention or reduction of radiation-induced immune suppression by the administration of immune stimulants before or during radiotherapy. BCG (Sparks *et al.*, 1974), Levamisole (Ramot *et al.*, 1976), C. parvum (Milas, 1974), thymosine (Hardy *et al.*, 1976), transfer factor (Order *et al.*, 1974), zymosan (Forsberg *et al.*, 1959), endotoxins (Smith *et al.*, 1957) and mixed bacterial toxins (Cole *et al.*, 1966) have all been considered in this context. If the results of *in vitro* studies are considered to reflect accurately the situation *in vivo* this approach may produce practical results by permitting the continuance of present radiotherapy regimes with much reduced immune suppression. Pretreatment has generally been found more effective than treatment after radiotherapy.

The Effects of Chemotherapy

Most, if not all, agents used in the chemotherapy of cancer cause readily identifiable alterations in lymphocyte and macrophage numbers and affect their function *in vitro* and *in vivo*, as indicated by the occurrence of opportunistic infections (Levine *et al.*, 1972; Simone *et al.*, 1972). The literature on the effects of the numerous and increasing range of cytotoxic agents available and their seemingly endless combinations on the immunological system is vast. A detailed review is beyond the scope of this book and the interested reader should refer to articles such as that by Leventhal *et al.* (1974).

I have confined my comments to a consideration of established general principles which are likely to be of importance in considering the effect of these agents on the host-tumour interaction.

It has been known for many years that chemotherapeutic agents depress immunological function in experimental animals. That cell-mediated immunity may be depressed was shown by a poor response to DNCB in guinea pigs receiving 6-mercaptopurine, actinomycin-D or Vinkaleuko-blastine (Maguire and Maibach, 1961) and by depression of the graft versus host reaction in mice receiving cytotoxic drugs (Owens and Santos, 1971). Depressed humoral responsiveness was indicated by a poor response to TAB vaccination by mice receiving cytotoxic agents (Berenbaum, 1962), reduced production of antibodies cytotoxic to SRBC by rats similarly treated (Santos and Owens, 1964) and poor antibody production by guinea pigs receiving cyclophosphamide, azathioprine or 5-fluorouracil (Maibach and Maguire, 1966).

In man, chemotherapy associated leucopenia and lymphopenia are well recognised complications of most agents and regimes (Bodey *et al.*, 1966; Green and Borella, 1973; Graham-Pole *et al.*, 1975). Immunoglobulin and antibody production is generally depressed and the capacity to produce antibody in response to primary or recall antigens is impaired (Dupuy *et al.*, 1971; Borella and Webster, 1971). Cell mediated immunity is also generally depressed (Hersh and Oppenheim, 1967; Ohno and Hersh, 1970; Campbell *et al.*, 1973), but it is of note that specific responsiveness to antigenic stimulation is slower to recover after the cessation of chemotherapy than are non-specific lymphocyte responses to mitogens (Green and Borella, 1973). The response to an encounter with a new antigen is more affected than is restimulation of an already established delayed hypersensitivity response (Hersh *et al.*, 1971; Dupuy *et al.*, 1971). Studies of the cells affected by chemotherapy indicate depression of B and T lymphocytes and macrophages (Leventhal *et al.*, 1974). Most authors have reported B lymphocytes to be more affected than T lymphocytes except where steroids have been the agent employed. There has been speculation that this selective pattern of immune depression may reduce blocking antibody production and so predispose to a favourable outcome (Griswold *et al.*, 1972; Mott, 1973). There are reports of the disappearance of blocking activity after chemotherapy (Sinkovics *et al.*, 1972) but this interesting suggestion remains unproved. Chemotherapy is also reported to reduce severely the number of detectable K cells in the blood (Campbell *et al.*, 1973).

The severity and duration of the effect induced varies with the agents used and the dose, rhythm and duration of treatment. Cycle active agents affect cells in mitosis and premitosis (Winkelstein, 1973) while non-cycle active agents may also affect intermitotic cells. This may partly explain the disparity between results obtained with tests involving proliferation and mitosis (blastogenesis assays), and those from tests such as MIF production, interferon production and plaque assays involving intermitotic cells (Möller and Möller, 1965; Bloom *et al.*, 1972; Rocklin, 1973; Wallen *et al.*, 1973). It has also been shown that various cytotoxic drugs are selectively active against specific lymphocyte subpopulations. Cyclophosphamide, for instance, is more active against B lymphocytes than T lymphocytes (Lerman and Weidanz, 1970; Turk and Poulter, 1972; Stockman *et al.*, 1973).

In contrast to the major prolonged alterations of lymphocyte populations and function seen after radiotherapy, the effects of chemotherapy measured *in vitro* in this way seem less severe and distinctly transient (Zweiman and Phillips, 1970; Sen and Borella, 1973; Green and Borella, 1973; Campbell *et al.*, 1973). Nonetheless it has to be conceded that infective complications of chemotherapy, including opportunistic infections are markedly more troublesome and frequent than those associated with radiotherapy. As expected, treatment duration and drug dosage are important in determining the extent of chemotherapy linked morbidity. High dosage inductive chemotherapy, often with combinations of agents, designed to bring a patient into remission induces marked immunesuppression (Campbell *et al.*, 1973) while lower dose maintenance schedules are associated with more minor effects *in vivo* and *in vitro* (Borella and Webster, 1971; Jones *et al.*, 1971). An interesting phenomenon known as immunological rebound or overshoot has been identified as occurring during the ten to twenty days which follow cessation of chemotherapy. Immunological parameters, depressed during chemotherapy have been found to return to *and exceed* pretreatment levels. This has been observed with the response to recall antigens (Cheema and Hersh, 1971; Harris and Stewart, 1972; Leventhal *et al.*, 1974), to transplantation antigens (Harris and Stewart, 1972) and tumour-associated antigens (Leventhal *et al.*, 1972) and with E-rosetting cells (T lymphocytes) (Serrou and Dubois, 1975). It is claimed that strong immunological rebound indicates a good prognosis (Cheema and Hersh, 1971; Harris and Stewart, 1972) and it may be that immunological stimulation during this period will be especially effective.

Chemotherapy has been associated with the induction of malignant disease. This has been observed with chemotherapy for malignant tumours (Spykens-Smit and Meyler, 1970; Kyle *et al.*, 1970; Rosner and Grünwald, 1974), for renal disease with or without the presence of a renal allograft (Fahey, 1971; Roberts and Bell, 1976) and for autoimmune disease (Tannenbaum and Schur, 1974; Westberg and Swolin, 1976). As with radiotherapy the most important mechanism is likely to be agent induced mutagenesis, but depressed immune activity against emerging neoplastic clones or oncogenic viruses cannot be excluded.

Immunological depression by chemotherapeutic agents may be combatted by judicious immune stimulation and it has been claimed that the beneficial effect of BCG immune stimulation in certain leukaemias may be mediated in this way.

Other Factors

Immunosuppressive activities must not be assigned to surgery, radiotherapy or chemotherapy without considering the many other factors which may be partly responsible for a decline in lymphocyte numbers and function. Drugs such as steroids (Claman, 1972; Yu *et al.*, 1974), including those used as contraceptives (Hagen and Froland, 1972; Fitzgerald *et al.*, 1973), antibiotics (Zwaveling, 1962; Gaylarde and Sarkany, 1972), anti-convulsants (Grob and Herold, 1972) and sedatives can modify lymphocyte activities. Concomitant conditions such as pregnancy (Finn *et al.*, 1972; Purtillo *et al.*, 1972; Walker *et al.*, 1972), nutritional deficiency and anaemia (Joynson *et al.*, 1972; Bhaskaram and Reddy, 1975; MacDougall *et al.*, 1975; Srikantia *et al.*, 1976), uraemia and liver failure may also be significant. Interest has recently been shown in the possible effects of psychological stress on the immune response and the indications are that cell-mediated immunity may be depressed by situations such as bereavement (Bartrop *et al.*, 1977) and major stressful undertakings such as those involved in aerospace travel (Kimzey, 1974).

References

Alexander, P. (1976) *Int. J. Rad. Oncol. Biol. Phys.* **1**, 369.
Bancewicz, J., Gray, A. and Lindop, G. (1973). *Brit. J. Surg.* **60**, 314.
Bartrop, R. W., Luckhurst, E., Lazarus, L., Kiloh, L. G. and Penny, R. (1977). *Lancet* **1**, 834.
Berenbaum, M. C. (1962). *Biochem. Pharmacol.* **11**, 29.
Berenbaum, M. C., Fluck, P. A. and Hurst, N. P. (1973). *Brit. J. exp. Path.* **54**, 597.
Bhaskaram, C. and Reddy, V. (1975). *Brit. med. J.* **3**, 522.
Blomgren, H., Wasserman, J. and Littbrand, B. (1974). *Acta Radiol.* **13**, 357.
Blomgren, H., Glas, U. and Melen, B. (1974a). *Acta Radiol. (Ther.)* **13**, 185.
Blomgren, H., Wasserman, J. and Littbrand, B. (1974b). *Acta Radiol. (Ther.)* **13**, 357.
Blomgren, H., Berg, R., Wasserman, J. and Glas, U. (1976). *Int. J. Rad. Oncol. Biol. Phys.* **1**, 177.
Bloom, B. R., Gaffney, J. and Jimenez, L. (1972). *J. Immunol.* **109**, 1395.
Bodey, G. P., Buckley, M., Sathe, Y. S. and Freireich, E. J. (1966). *Ann. int. Med.* **64**, 328.
Borella, L. and Webster, R. G. (1971). *Cancer Res.* **31**, 420.
Brown, A. M., Lally, E. T., Frankel, A., Harwick, R., Davis, L. W. and Rominger, C. J. (1975). *Cancer* **35**, 1154.
Bruce, D. L. and Wingard, D. N. (1971). *Anesthesiology* **34**, 271.
Buinauskas, P., Brown, E. R. and Cole, W. H. (1965). *J. Surg. Res.* **5**, 538.
Buckston, K. E., Court Brown, W. M. and Smith, D. G. (1967). *Nature* **214**, 470.
Campbell, A. C., Hersey, P., MacLennan, I. C. M., Kay, H. E. M., Pike, M. C. and the Medical Research Council's Working Party on Leukaemia in Childhood (1973). *Brit. med. J.* **2**, 385.
Check, J. H., Damsker, J. I., Brady, L. W. and O'Neill, E. A. (1973). *Cancer* **32**, 580.
Chee, C. A., Ilbery, P. L. T. and Rickinson, A. B. (1974). *Brit. J. Radiol.* **47**, 37.
Cheema, A. R. and Hersh, E. M. (1971). *Cancer Res.* **28**, 851.
Claman, H. N. (1972). *New Engl. J. Med.* **287**, 388.
Clements, J. A. and Kramer, S. (1974). *Cancer* **34**, 193.
Cochran, A. J., Spilg, W. G. S., Mackie, R. M. and Thomas, C. E. (1972). *Brit. med. J.* **4**, 67.
Cole, D. R., Dreyer, B., Rousselot, L. M. and Tendler, M. D. (1966). *Amer. J. Roent. Radium Ther. and Nuclear Med.* **47**, 997.
Constantian, M. B., Menzdian, J. O., Nimberg, R. B., Schmid, K. and Mannick, J. A. (1975). *Clin. Res.* **23**, 410A.
Cooper, A. J., Irvine, J. M. and Turnbull, A. R. (1974). *Immunology* **27**, 393.
Court Brown, W. and Doll, R. (1957). *Spec. Rep. Ser. Med. Res. Council* **295.**
Dubois, J. B., Serrou, B. and Pourquier, H. (1975). *Bull. du Cancer* **62**, 1.
Dupuy, J. M., Kourilsky, F. M., Fradelizzi, D., Feingold, N., Jacquillat, C., Bernard, J. and Dausset, J. (1971). *Cancer* **27**, 323.
Einhorn, N., Henle, G., Henle, W., Klein, G. and Clifford, P. (1972). *Int. J. Cancer* **9**, 182.

Engesett, A., Froland, S. S., Brenner, K. and Host, H. (1973). *Scand. J. Haematol.* **11**, 195.

Espanol, T., Todd, G. B. and Soothill, J. F. (1974). *Clin. exp. Immunol.* **18**, 73.

Fahey, J. L. (1971). *Ann. intern. Med.* **75**, 310.

Finn, R., St. Hill, C. A., Govan, A. J., Ralfs, I. G. and Gurney, F. J. (1972). *Brit. med. J.* **3**, 160.

Fitzgerald, P. H., Pickering, A. F. and Ferguson, D. N. (1973). *Lancet* **1**, 616.

Forsberg, A., Lingen, C., Ernster, L. and Lindberg, O. (1959). *Exper. Cell Res.* **16**, 7.

Gaylarde, P. M. and Sarkany, I. (1972). *Brit. med. J.* **3**, 144.

Ghossein, N. A., Bosworth, J. L. and Bases, R. E. (1975). *Cancer* **35**, 1616.

Goswitz, F. A., Andrews, G. A. and Kriseley, R. M. P. (1963). *Blood* **21**, 605.

Graham-Pole, J., Willoughby, M. L. N., Aitken, S. and Ferguson, A. (1975). *Brit. med. J.* **2**, 467.

Green, A. A. and Borella, L. (1973). *Blood* **42**, 99.

Griswold, D. E., Heppner, G. M. and Calabresi, P. (1972). *Cancer Res.* **32**, 298.

Grob, P. J. and Herold, G. E. (1972). *Brit. med. J.* **2**, 561.

Gross, L., Manfredi, D. L. and Protos, A. (1973). *Radiology* **106**, 653.

Hagen, C. and Froland, A. (1972). *Lancet* **1**, 1185.

Hall, E. E. (1973). "Radiobiology for the Radiologists." Harper and Row, Hagerstown, Md.

Han, T. (1972). *Lancet* **1**, 742.

Hardy, M. A., Oattner, A. M., Sarkan, D. K., Stoffer, J. A. and Friedmann, N. (1976). *Cancer* **37**, 98.

Harris, J. E. and Stewart, T. H. M. (1972). *In* "Proceedings of the Sixth Leucocyte Culture Conference" (Schwarz, M. R., Ed.) 555. Academic Press, New York and London.

Heier, H. E., Christensen, I., Froland, S. S. and Engeset, A. (1975). *Lymphology* **8**, 69.

Hempelmann, L. H. (1968). *Science* **160**, 163.

Hersh, E. M., Whitecar, J. P., McCredie, K. B., Bodey, G. P. and Freireich, E. J. (1971). *New Engl. J. Med.* **285**, 1211.

Hersh, E. M. and Oppenheim, J. J. (1967). *Cancer Res.* **27**, 98.

Howard, R. J. and Simmons, R. L. (1974). *Surg. Gynec. Obstet.* **139**, 771.

Humphrey, L. J., Amerson, J. R. and Frederickson, E. L. (1970). *Anesth. and Analg.* **49**, 809.

Humphrey, G. B., Nesbit, M. E., Chary, K. K. N. and Krivit, W. (1972). *Cancer* **29**, 402.

Ilbery, P. L. T., Rickinson, A. B. and Thrum, C. E. (1971). *Brit. J. Radiol.* **44**, 834.

Jones, L. H., Hardisty, R. M., Wells, D. G. and Kay, H. E. M. (1971). *Brit. med. J.* **4**, 329.

Joynson, D. H. M., Jacobs, A., Murraywalker, D. and Dolby, A. E. (1972). *Lancet* **2**, 1058.

Kimzey, S. L. (1974). *Acta Astronautica* **127**, 1.

Kyle, R. A., Pierre, R. V. and Bayard, E. D. (1970). *New Engl. J. Med.* **283**, 1121.

Leguit, P., Meinesz, A., Zeijlemaker, W. D., Schellerens, P. T. A. and Eijsvoogel, V. P. (1973). *Int. Arch. Allergy Appl. Immun.* **44**, 101.

Lerman, S. P. and Weidanz, W. P. (1970). *J. Immunol.* **105**, 614.

Leventhal, B. G., Cohen, P. and Triem, S. C. (1974). *In* "Immunological parameters of host-tumor relationships" (Weiss, D. Ed.) Vol. 3, 52-73. Academic Press, New York and London.

Levine, A. S., Graw, R. G. and Young, R. C. (1972). *Sem. Haematol.* **9**, 141.

Mackie, R. M., Spilg, W. G. S., Thomas, C. E. and Cochran, A. J. (1972). *Br. J. Derm.* **87,** 523.

Maguire, H. C. and Maibach, H. I. (1961). *J. Invest. Dermatol.* **37,** 427.

Maibach, H. I. and Maguire, H. C. (1966). *Int. Arch. Allerg.* **29,** 209.

Meyer, K. K., Machler, G. L. and Beck, W. C. (1973). *Arch. Surg.* **107,** 159.

Milas, L. (1974). "Interaction of radiation and host immune defense mechanisms in malignancy." 293-313. Brookhaven National Laboratory.

Millard, R. E. (1965). *J. Clin. Path.* **18,** 783.

Möller, E. and Möller, G. (1965). *Nature* **208,** 260.

Mott, M. G. (1973). *Lancet* **1,** 1092.

Munster, A. M., Eurenius, K., Mortensen, R. F. and Mason, A. D. (1972). *Transplantation* **14,** 106.

Munster, A. M. and Artz, C. P. S. (1974). *Med. J. Nashville* **67,** 935.

Munster, A. M. (1976). *Lancet* **1,** 1329.

McCoy, J. L., Jerome, L. F., Dean, J. H., Perlin, E., Oldham, R. K., Char, D. H., Cohen, M. H., Felix, E. L. and Herberman, R. B. (1975). *J. nat. Cancer Inst.* **55,** 19.

McCredie, J. A., Inch, W. R. and Sutherland, R. M. (1972). *Cancer* **29,** 349.

MacDougall, L. G., Anderson, R., McNab, G. M. and Katz, J. (1975). *J. Pediat.* **86,** 833.

Nunn, J. F., Sharp, J. A. and Kimball, K. L. (1970). *Nature* **226,** 85.

Ohno, R. and Hersh, E. M. (1970). *Blood* **35,** 250.

Order, S. E., Donahue, V. and Knapp, R. (1974). *In* "Interaction of radiation and host immune defense mechanisms in malignancy." 363-378. Brookhaven National Laboratory.

Owens, A. H. and Santos, G. W. (1971). *Transplantation* **11,** 378.

Park, S. K., Brody, J. I., Wallace, H. A. and Blakemore, N. S. (1971). *Lancet* **1,** 53.

Purtillo, D. T., Hallgren, H. M. and Yunis, E. J. (1972). *Lancet* **1,** 769.

Ramot, B., Binaminov, M., Shoham, C. H. and Rosenthal, E. (1976). *New Engl. J. Med.* **294,** 809.

Riddle, P. R. and Berenbaum, M. C. (1967). *Lancet* **1,** 746.

Roberts, M. M. and Bell, R. (1976). *Lancet* **2,** 768.

Rocklin, R. E. (1973). *In* "Proceedings of the Seventh Leucocyte Culture Conference." (F. Daguillard, ed.) 381. Academic Press, New York and London.

Rosner, F. and Grünwald, H. (1974). *Amer. J. Med.* **57,** 927.

Rubin, P., Landman, S., Moyer, E., Keller, B. and Cicclo, S. (1973). *Cancer* **32,** 699.

Santos, G. W. and Owens, A. H. (1964). *Bull. Johns Hopk. Hosp.* **114,** 384.

Schoenenberger, G. H., Burkhardt, F., Kalberer, F., Muller, W., Stadtler, K., Vogt, P. and Allgöwer, M. (1975). *Surg. Gynec. Obstet.* **141,** 555.

Sen, L. and Borella, L. (1973). *Cell Immunol.* **9,** 84.

Serrou, B. and Dubois, J. B. (1975).

Simone, J. V., Holland, E. and Johnson, W. (1972). *Blood* **39,** 759.

Sinkovics, J. G., Cabiness, J. R. and Shullenberger, C. C. (1972). *Cancer* **30,** 1428.

Slater, J. M., Ngo, E. and Lau, B. H. S. (1976). *Am. J. Roentgenol.* **126,** 313.

Smith, W. W., Alderman, I. M. and Gillespie, R. E. (1957). *Amer. J. Physiol.* **191,** 124-130.

Sokal, J. E. and Firat, D. (1965). *Amer. J. Med.* **39,** 452.

Sparks, F. C., Eilber, F. R., Holmes, E. C. and Morton, D. L. (1974). *In* "Interaction of radiation and host immune defense mechanisms in malignancy." 314-322. Brookhaven National Laboratory.

Spykens-Smit, C. G. and Meyler, L. (1970). *Lancet* **2,** 671.

Srikantia, S. G., Siva Prasad, J., Bhaskaram, C. and Krishnamachari, Kaur (1976). *Lancet* **1**, 1307.
Stjernswärd, J. (1972). *Ann. Inst. Pasteur* **122**, 883.
Stjernswärd, J., Jondal, M., Vanky, F., Wigzell, H. and Sealy, R. (1972). *Lancet* **2**, 1352.
Stockman, G. D., Heim, L. R., South, M. A. and Trentin, J. J. (1973). *J. Immunol.* **110**, 285.
Stratton, J. A., Byfield, P. E., Byfield, J. A. *et al.* (1975). *J. Clin. Invest.* **56**, 88.
Suter, G. M. (1947). *USAEC Document* **MDDC** 824.
Tannenbaum, H. and Schur, P. H. (1974). *Arthritis Rheum.* **17**, 15.
Thomas, J. M., Coy, P., Lewis, H. S. and Yuen, A. (1971). *Cancer* **27**, 1046.
Turk, J. L. and Poulter, L. W. (1972). *Clin. exp. Immunol.* **10**, 285.
Vasudevan, D. M., Balakrishnan, K. and Talwar, G. P. (1971). *Indian J. Med. Res.* **59**, 1653.
Viljanen, M. K., Kanito, J., Vapaavori, M. and Torvanen, P. (1973). *Brit. med. J.* **3**, 499.
Vose, B. M. and Moudgil, G. C. (1975). *Brit. med. J.* **1**, 56.
Vose, B. M. and Moudgil, G. C. (1976). *Immunology* **30**, 123.
Walker, J. S., Freeman, C. B. and Harris, R. (1972). *Brit. med. J.* **3**, 469.
Wallen, W. C., Dean, J. H. and Lucas, D. O. (1973). *Cellular Immunology* **6**, 110.
Westberg, N. G. and Swolin, B. (1976). *Acta med. Scand.* **199**, 373.
Wingard, D. W., Lang, R. and Humphrey, L. J. (1967). *J. Surg. Res.* **7**, 430.
Winkelstein, A. (1973). *J. Clin. Invest.* **52**, 2293.
Wohl, H. and Ghossein, N. A. (1971). *Oncology* **25**, 344.
Yu, D. T. Y., Clements, P. J., Paulus, H. E., Peter, J. B., Levy, J. and Barnett, E. V. (1974). *J. Clin. Invest.* **53**, 565.
Zwaveling, A. (1962). *Cancer* **15**, 790.
Zweimann, B. and Phillips, S. M. (1970). *Science* **160**, 1395.

8

Immunotherapy

Even if it is a medieval form of therapy, it works
Georges Mathé, 1976

The results of conventional therapy indicate that new approaches are urgently required, especially in the treatment of metastatic malignancy. For example patients who present with a primary melanoma without evidence of spread, have a 5 year survival rate around 80%, and approaching 100% for superficial, thin tumours of favourable histogenetic type. Patients with metastases in the regional lymph nodes, either in combination with a primary at initial presentation, or subsequent to treatment of a primary have a 5 year survival rate around 20% and those with visceral spread only exceptionally survive for more than one year (Cochran, 1969). Surgical management of the early patient is often very satisfactory, but neither surgery nor radiotherapy nor chemotherapy provide an acceptable frequency of cure in the patient with significantly spread disease.

Not even the most committed supporters of immunotherapy would claim that, as presently practised, it offers a dramatic answer to the management of patients with metastatic cancer. It may be that techniques, as yet unimagined, will make our attempts at immunotherapy seem quite inappropriate. However the techniques and enthusiasms for investigating immunotherapy are currently available and even if the therapeutic materials are crude and our understanding of their pharmacology minimal, the scale of the clinical problem demands adequate investigation of the power and applicability of immune therapy.

The harnessing of the impressive destructive capacities of the immune response for cancer therapy has always been a major goal for tumour immunologists. Ideally this chapter would be the high point of the book and would describe major extensions of survival or, better still, cancer cure by immunotherapy. In fact it can be no more than a situation report which shows that by using crude weapons, pragmatic timing and probably facile tactics against a poorly identified and subtle enemy some small victories have been recorded for immunotherapy. The lessons learned have clarified some specific theoretical and practical characteristics of ideal immunological reagents and those situations in which malignancy is likely to be most susceptible to immunological attack, either alone or as part of a combined modality approach. These achievements, while small in the context of the eventual aims, are nonetheless significant.

While the past decade has seen increasing interest in immune manipulation as part of the treatment of cancer the philosophy which has led to attempts at "immunotherapy" is of considerably greater antiquity. Cancer regression in association with bacterial infections and inflammatory processes has been recorded for many years. Most such reports are to some degree anecdotal but taken together they make a reasonably persuasive case for a (fortuitously) beneficial effect of some infections on malignant disease (Nauts et al., 1953; Sensenig et al., 1963; Takita, 1970). It is also claimed that there is an inverse relationship between the incidence of cancer and the incidence of infections (Jacobsen, 1934). Stern (1971) postulated that the reticuloendothelial system activated by microorganismal stimulation may also be more active in cancer prevention or in inducing regression of established tumours and Burchenal (1966) suggested that the response of African Burkitt lymphoma patients to low dose chemotherapy might be due to an infection stimulated reticuloendothelial system. These observations and suggestions, while clearly of great interest, must not be accepted as indicating that all microorganismal infections cause reticuloendothelial stimulation. There is, for instance, evidence that virus infections of animals (Salaman, 1969) and man (vonPirquet, 1908; Starr and Berkovitch, 1964) and even the administration of a virus vaccine such as that used against measles (Mellman and Wetton, 1963; Brody and McAlister, 1964) may be immunosuppressive. Plasmodial infections are also immune depressant in mice (Wedderburn, 1970).

Reticuloendothelial stimulation associated with some infections certainly justifies the search for microorganisms and microorganismal products which provide an acceptable stimulus to the reticuloendothelial system. Such agents might be valuable in the prevention of cancer in high risk groups and the control of metastases in tumour bearing patients. Early work of this kind was undertaken by William B. Coley in New York and various workers in Germany during the latter years of the 19th century and the early part of the 20th century (Coley, 1891; Coley, 1893; Nauts et al., 1946). Coley induced erysipelas by streptococcal infection and later, because of the difficulty and dangers of employing live vaccines (present day therapists will sympathise with his dilemma) sterilised streptococcal cultures and finally filtered material from a variety of microbial sources (Coley's toxins). Interest in this type of approach has been maintained over the intervening years by a small band of dedicated enthusiasts and not inconsiderable successes are documented (see Nauts et al., 1953 for review).

Interest in the use of streptococcal and other bacterial preparations continues and the extensive current interest in agents such as Bacillus Calmette-Guérin (BCG), Corynebacterium parvum (CP) and vaccinia virus may be regarded as an extension of the early interest in microorganismal products as stimulators of the reticuloendothelial system.

General Considerations

TYPES OF IMMUNOTHERAPY

Depending upon their interpretation of the experimental and clinical evidence immunotherapists divide readily into two groups. There are those who believe that the immune reaction spontaneously induced *in vivo* by tumour associated antigens is potentially tumour destructive, but in its naturally occurring state is generally too weak to induce regression or is relatively weak in the face of coexisting influences such as blocking factors. If this is the case then *all* that is required to permit the amplification of the response to an effective level is to boost it or modify it to shift the balance against the production of blocking or other deleterious activity. This might be achieved by general stimulation of the reticuloendothelial (RE) system (*active non-specific immunotherapy*) or might require secondary immunisation against TAA to which a weak reaction already exists or the raising of a new immune response to TAA which have not spontaneously induced an immune response (*active specific immunotherapy*). This second approach would seem specially appropriate where an immune response to tumour antigens is directed against tumour associated antigens which do not have a rejection inducing potential or which, while displayed in early tumour development are modulated, genetically suppressed or masked later in the disease. Both the above approaches employ the systemic administration of adjuvants and/or immunogenic materials from tumour cells. A related and practical approach to the control of localised accessible disease is the application of sensitising agents such as DNCB or DNFB to tumours or the injection of immune stimulants such as BCG, CP or vaccinia virus into tumours (*local immunotherapy*). The induced delayed hypersensitivity reaction destroys the tumour cells, apparently *en passant* although it is possible that release of tumour antigen after tumour cell breakdown induces specific immunisation and adds an element of active specific immunotherapy, which may explain the regression of a minority of tumour nodules remote from the treated area.

A second group of immunotherapists work on the assumption that the anti-tumour immune response, while indicative of the existence of tumour antigens and their interactions with the host RE system, has no significant tumour rejecting capacity in the overwhelming majority of situations. If this is the case active immunotherapy is inappropriate and can only magnify an interesting but irrelevant epiphenomenon. The need is to raise anti-tumour reagents in other members of the same species or members of other species who recognise and react to the relatively unique characteristics of the tumour cells. Such reagents could then be administered to tumour patients (*passive immunotherapy*). The most obvious materials for use in this way are humoral antibodies and specifically sensitised lymphocytes, but there is also interest in the transfer of information by administering substances such as "immune" RNA or transfer factor from individuals with regressed tumour or who have been immunised to a tumour.

While it is easy to sub-divide the various forms of immunotherapy in this way it is possible that effective regimes will require the skilful combination of different forms of therapy in sequence, the techniques to be employed being decided by the volume of tumour present, its growth or regression and the patient's immune competence.

LOGISTIC CONSIDERATIONS IN IMMUNOTHERAPY

The employment of immunotherapy has been largely empirical and we urgently require information on the best agents to employ, their optimum doses and the most appropriate routes and timings of their administration. It seems most unlikely that immunotherapy will *replace* traditional methods of therapy, however, appropriately combined, it may be a valuable adjunct to standard therapy and we urgently need to assess the usefulness of immuno-chemotherapy and combinations of irradiation therapy and immunotherapy. On available evidence the morbidity of immunotherapy has been only moderate and mortality extremely low, however we need much more information on the complications of each agent or combination of agents.

While most of these questions remain to be answered, certain general principles have emerged from the studies undertaken to the present.

Timing of immunotherapy in relation to tumour volume

There is considerable evidence that immunotherapy is maximally effective against a relatively small number of tumour cells and should probably be confined to patients with little or no clinically detectable disease, in fact the period after tumour reduction by conventional therapy (Fig. 8.1A). This ideally would be immediately after primary therapy in high risk tumours and after treatment of the first recurrence in others. Trials of immunotherapy of patients with this "susceptible" stage of disease have only recently been undertaken as immunotherapists have (properly) faced the conventional limitations placed on those attempting to exploit a new therapeutic approach. Immunotherapy was therefore initially confined to patients with advanced disease (Fig. 8.1B), who were unlikely to respond to conventional therapy. It is perhaps not surprising that these patients showed little or no response to any form of immune therapy in the great majority of cases. It is therefore the absence of major problems of therapy-linked morbidity and mortality rather than clear therapeutic effectiveness which has emboldened therapists to treat patients with less advanced disease.

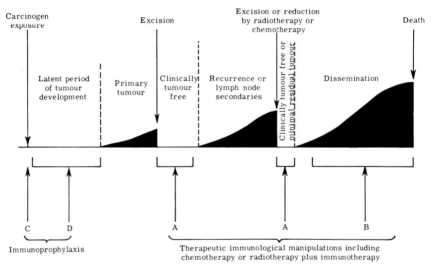

Fig. 8.1. The timing of immunotherapy.
A. Therapeutic immunological manipulation when clinically detectable tumour is absent or minimal. B. Therapeutic immunological manipulation when tumour burden is considerable. A and B may be combined with radiation therapy or chemotherapy. C. Immunoprophylaxis. Immune manipulation at time of carcinogen exposure or (in animals) at time of tumour transplantation. D. Immunoprophylaxis. Immune manipulation during latent period between carcinogen exposure (or tumour transplantation) and emergence of a clinically detectable tumour.

Studies of timing of therapy have been hindered by the lack of animal models which closely resemble the growth kinetics and metastatic behaviour of spontaneous human tumours. In animal studies employing transplantable tumours it has proved relatively simple to prevent or retard tumour growth by administering adjuvants with or without tumour cell preparations prior to or at the same time as carcinogen exposure or tumour transplantation (Fig. 8.1C) or during the latent period prior to tumour development (Fig. 8.1D). It is difficult to see the relevance of this effect to human tumours unless this "immunoprophylaxis" were applicable to *carcinoma-in-situ* or to patients known to have had exposure to high concentrations of carcinogen*. Attempts to treat established spontaneous or transplanted tumours in animals (a situation slightly more reminiscent of that in man) have been markedly less successful.

Timing of immunotherapy in relation to other forms of therapy

The periods of immune suppression following radiotherapy, chemotherapy and surgery would seem best avoided from a strictly immunological standpoint when planning active immunotherapy. It has, however, been claimed that the administration of an adjuvant prior to or during potentially immune suppressive therapy will reduce the degree of suppression both of the immune response and of haemopoiesis. On the one hand this protective effect will reduce the incidence of opportunistic infections and problems of coagulation failure and on the other may allow the use of a dose of radiation or chemotherapy in excess of that normally possible. A further consideration is that immune stimulation may best be administered with chemotherapy at the time of post-depression "immunological overshoot" when the immune system seems especially responsive to stimulation.

Determination of dose, timing and frequency of administration of agents

The general principles devised for the testing of new chemotherapeutic agents should be followed (Carter and Slavik, 1975). There is no reason why immunological reagents should be excused the rigorous scrutiny accorded to other drugs.

Site and route of administration of immunotherapeutic agents

This is largely determined by the site and known degree of dissemination of tumour cells and is limited by toxicity and (in the case of living organisms) by problems of infection. Where a tumour has an obvious group of lymph nodes into which lymphatic spread is likely to occur it is arguable that stimulation of these nodes by judicious placing of immune stimulation may lead to the death of entrapped tumour cells.

Host immunocompetence

Therapeutic success with immunotherapy is claimed to be limited to patients who are immunocompetent prior to treatment or who develop competence during therapy (Hersh *et al.*, 1974). This seems to me a critical observation

---

*Claims that BCG, given as tuberculosis prophylaxis, may reduce the incidence of leukaemia in recipient children (Davignon *et al.*, 1970; Rosenthal *et al.*, 1972) remain to be substantiated (Comstock *et al.*, 1971; MRC, 1972). It has even been suggested that recipients may have an increase in lymphomas (Comstock *et al.*, 1975).

and it is unfortunate that the technology for assessing significant immuno-incompetence and our appreciation of what constitutes a significant level of abnormality remain far from complete. Regrettably, relatively few immuno-therapy studies have employed immunological competence as an inclusion or stratification criterion.

Selectivity of immune stimulation

If the theory which imputes "good" antitumour activity to cell-mediated immunity and "bad" blocking-type activity to at least some anti-tumour antibodies is correct, the ideal immunostimulants will selectively stimulate cellular immunity. This remains the working hypothesis but its foundations have undeniably been weakened by the demonstration of potentially favourable activities for antibodies such as in antibody-dependent, cell-mediated cytotoxicity (Chapter 3).

The reagents to be employed

It is now clear that different preparations of adjuvants such as BCG and CP vary widely in their physical, chemical and cultural characteristics, in their capacity to affect lymphocytes and macrophages *in vitro* and in their capacity to affect tumour growth and spread in animal models. We need to know much more of the significance of these variations and which parameters measurable *in vitro* predict anti-tumour activity *in vivo*.

Reagents to be used for passive immunotherapy should be as highly specific in their anti-tumour activity as is technically possible.

Interpretation of results

Positive anti-tumour activity and deleterious side effects, including tumour enhancement can only be identified by comparing the various regimes in concurrently controlled prospective clinical trials. With the possible exception of local immunotherapy there is at present no clinical situation where immunotherapy is universally accepted as the treatment of choice and from a purely therapeutic standpoint the *ad hoc* administration of immunotherapy cannot be justified. I believe that the majority of tumour immunologists and oncologists would agree with this statement, although I recognise that some highly experienced therapists would regard it as an overstatement.

Recording of results

In order to avoid unnecessary duplication of studies it is desirable that negative results are reported and it is to be hoped that journal editors will see the desirability of this and continue to accept such papers for publication. It is desirable too, that side effects be recorded as rapidly as possible and not merely as confirmatory comments after oral presentations at meetings.

A More Detailed Consideration of the Different Types of Immunotherapy

ACTIVE IMMUNOTHERAPY

Active non-specific immunotherapy

The requirement here is for a strong stimulant of the immunological apparatus, which carries no major side effects or morbidity and which on present evidence should probably preferentially stimulate cell mediated immunity. The agents employed divide readily into biological agents, whole micro-organisms or materials derived from them, and synthetic preparations. The majority of studies to the present have employed biological adjuvants, but there is increasing interest in synthetic materials such as Levamisole and poly-IC.

Bacillus Calmette-Guérin (BCG). This attenuated bovine tubercle bacillus is the biological adjuvant which has received most attention thus far.

Early studies indicated that an infection with virulent *Mycobacterium tuberculosis* was associated with an increase in strength of humoral immunity (Lewis and Loomis, 1924) and cell-mediated immunity (Dienes, 1936). Subsequently it has been shown that exposure to mycobacterial materials causes wide ranging effects *in vivo*. These include increased resistance to unrelated organisms (Dubois and Schaedler, 1957), increased strength of allograft rejection (Balner *et al.*, 1962) and increased resistance to tumour challenge (Biozzi *et al.*, 1954; Old *et al.*, 1961; Baldwin and Pimm, 1973). Alterations *in vitro* include increased phagocytosis (Biozzi *et al.*, 1954), the development of macrophages capable of killing tumour cells (Hibbs *et al.*, 1972; Evans and Alexander, 1972; Cleveland *et al.*, 1974), increased cell mediated immunity (Littman *et al.*, 1973; Mackaness *et al.*, 1974) and increased circulating T (E-rosetting) cells (Serrou *et al.*, 1975). An increase in mitogen responsiveness by lymphocytes has been recorded by some authors (Cohen *et al.*, 1974) but not by others (Gutterman *et al.*, 1973; Golub *et al.*, 1976).

These multiple and diverse observations are the basis of the continuing interest in mycobacteria and their products as immunological adjuvants.

The clinical applicability of a highly pathogenic micro-organism is limited and attempts have therefore been made to employ *M. tuberculosis* in an inactive or killed form. These achieved only limited success until Freund (1956) introduced a highly successful adjuvant consisting of heat killed mycobacteria emulsified in mineral oil. This however had the disadvantage of inducing severe necrosis at the injection site.

In view of the locally toxic properties of Freund's complete adjuvant attention was directed to exploitation of less damaging adjuvants, including

BCG. Biozzi et al. (1959) found BCG to have antitumour activity against the Erhlich ascites tumour in mice and Old et al. (1959) recorded similar activity against a transplantable mouse tumour. In the intervening years a plethora of reports has confirmed these early observations in many different tumour systems and species. In animal studies BCG has proved most active in immunoprophylaxis, against small numbers of tumour cells, when brought into close contact with tumour cells and when given in adequate dose as measured by the number of live bacteria administered.

Reports of the use of BCG against human cancer followed, initially in acute lymphoblastic leukaemia (Mathé et al., 1963) and then in other leukaemias and "haematosarcomas" (Mathé et al., 1967). Intense investigation of BCG in man dates from the late 1960s when Mathé recorded the results of BCG therapy in children with acute lymphoblastic leukaemia (Mathé et al., 1969). These children were brought into haematological remission by intensive chemotherapy and then divided into one group which received no further treatment and a second group which received maintenance therapy with BCG scarified weekly into the skin. The reported results were striking. The BCG recipients had a markedly lower incidence of relapse and some achieved remissions which have persisted to the present. All children in the group receiving no maintenance therapy relapsed. These findings were an enormous stimulus to further studies, and have recently been confirmed (EORTC, 1975, cited by Mathé 1976).

Other studies of BCG in the treatment of acute lymphoblastic leukaemia have not been successful. The British Medical Research Council Leukaemia Committee (1971) compared maintenance BCG with maintenance chemotherapy using methotrexate in acute lymphoblastic leukaemia and found BCG inferior to methotrexate in the maintenance of remissions. The reasons for the disparity between the Mathé study and the MRC study are unclear. There were differences between the trials in terms of the chemotherapy employed and the source, dosage and method of administration of BCG. Recent studies of BCG suggest that different preparations have different effects, including therapeutic effects, which appear to depend on characteristics of the mycobacteria, the method of culture employed in raising the vaccine, the proportion of living to dead intact mycobacteria and the amount of mycobacterial debris present (Halle-Pannenko et al., 1976). The reasons for the difference between the results of these two similar studies of BCG in acute lymphoblastic leukaemia, seem likely to remain a scientific conundrum. The effectiveness of combination chemotherapy in remission induction and maintenance has recently increased dramatically (although it is not without hazard—Aur et al., 1975) and most clinical haematologists now rely on this form of therapy rather than a combination of BCG and chemotherapy.

BCG has also been used in acute myeloblastic leukaemia (Crowther *et al.*, 1973; Freeman *et al.*, 1973; Vogler and Chan, 1974; Gutterman *et al.*, 1974). Most studies employed BCG with or without irradiated allogeneic tumour cells after remission induction by chemotherapy. Several studies suggested that immunotherapy treated patients had longer remissions than those maintained on chemotherapy alone, but the case for immunotherapy remains unproven in this disease. The use of different types of BCG, especially high viability preparations, or different routes and methods of application of BCG or the use of other immune stimulants may yield clearer clinical effect and it is to be hoped that controlled clinical trials of immunotherapy will continue in the leukaemias.

BCG has also been employed in the therapy of solid tumours, although such studies have been slower to develop and the utility of BCG in this situation remains to be established. For ethical reasons, most of the early trials concerned patients with relatively advanced disease and only recently has it been possible to investigate the effect of BCG in perpetuating the tumour free status or further reducing tumour burden after surgery or chemotherapy.

There are now a large number of clinical trials of BCG in many different types of solid tumour in progress as witnessed by the increasing bulk of the International Registry of Tumour Immunotherapy published by the U.S. National Institutes of Health. Most are still in progress and their results cannot yet be evaluated. Sadly the construction of some trials means that confident evaluation of their results will never be possible (Terry, 1978). Because of this it is clear that immunotherapy trials must conform to the simple but demanding rules governing the conduct of prospective, randomised, concurrently controlled, clinical trials.

Encouraging results have been obtained in melanoma by Bluming *et al.* (1972) who found high dose Pasteur strain BCG to prolong the disease free interval and increase survival.

Morton and his colleagues (1976) regard intralesional BCG as the treatment of choice in metastatic melanoma limited to the skin. The same authors gave BCG to melanoma patients with metastatic disease (Stages II and III) after excision of as much tumour as possible and benefits in terms of decreased recurrence rates and prolonged survival were observed. The trial was not randomised, nor concurrently controlled but the results were sufficiently encouraging to lead to the establishment of a currently active randomised clinical trial of BCG, after surgery in stage II and after surgery and chemotherapy in stage III. The Houston group from the M. D. Anderson Hospital have produced interesting data on the effects of BCG after surgical removal of melanomatous lymph nodes (Gutterman *et al.*, 1973), and of BCG combined with imidazole carboxamide chemotherapy in metastatic melanoma (Gutterman *et al.*, 1974). The impact of these studies is, however, lessened by the absence of concurrent control patients, the authors relying on historical groups.

Probably the most impressive recent report of BCG therapy is that by McKneally *et al.* (1976) who gave a single dose of BCG into the pleural cavity after lobectomy or pneumonectomy for lung cancer. In patients with limited tumour burden BCG dramatically reduced recurrences and improved survival relative to randomised control individuals who had no BCG. Given in this way BCG has *not* been beneficial in patients with more advanced disease. In a second randomised trial reported in the same issue of the Lancet, Pines (1976) found that BCG after radiotherapy for squamous carcinoma of lung prolonged survival during the first year of survival and reduced the incidence of peripheral metastases. That BCG can produce an effect in this most intransigent of cancers must be regarded as of major importance.*

It is a matter of major concern that we still know very little of the optima for dose, route of administration and timing of BCG and other adjuvants. In most animal experiments, relatively minor adjustments of an adjuvant regime may alter a tumour inhibitory effect to tumour enhancement. It is therefore possible that the adjuvants available would be markedly more effective if we could strike the correct regime for their administration. If it proves necessary painstakingly to examine all possible doses, routes and timings of BCG therapy, the task seems daunting and endless. The establishment of good animal models and the identification of BCG characteristics which may be simply examined *in vitro* and will predict therapeutic effectiveness is thus a matter of extreme urgency.

Mathé (1976) discusses these matters authoritatively and presents a suggested optimum dose for *fresh living Pasteur BCG*, a dose which differs for individuals showing immunocompetence to recall antigens and those in whom this type of reaction cannot be detected. He states that a "septicemia of a given intensity . . . correlated with the antitumour action" and, if these conclusions are correct, the need appears to be to establish a symbiosis between cancer patient and mycobacteria. On the basis of studies in mice and monkeys (Jurczyk-Procyk *et al.*, 1976) Mathé suggests reasonably that a precisely metered septicaemia could best be achieved by the intravenous administration of BCG. Given by this route in man BCG is well tolerated but may induce immune depression and tumour enhancement in allergic (immunocompetent) patients.

These bold and instructive studies present considerable problems. Fresh Institute Pasteur BCG is not readily available to most workers in the immunotherapy field and the data on doseage cannot be extrapolated directly to other strains and preparations of BCG. It is theoretically possible

---

*An attempt to repeat exactly McKneally's study has recently commenced with support from the British Medical Research Council.

that comparable data could be obtained for other BCG preparations, but few groups possess the facilities to undertake such studies. However, there is increasing demand for better characterisation of BCG and it may be that this will be the main direction of BCG research in the next few years.

Complications of BCG therapy are dealt with in a subsequent section. They have largely related to the use of a living infective organism and logically interest has been directed to identifying the materials within the organisms which mediate the adjuvant effect. A large number of myco-bacterial extracts have accordingly been prepared. The best known include "Methanol extracted residue" (Weiss, 1972), "hydrosoluble adjuvant" (Hiu, 1972) and "water soluble adjuvant" (Adam et al., 1972). While preparations of this type show some effects in vitro and in vivo in animals they remain at an early developmental stage and have not yet been tested extensively in man. Another related approach which has shown activity against animal tumours is the attachment of mycobacterial cell wall materials to mineral oil droplets (Ribi et al., 1966; Ribi et al., 1971; Zbar et al., 1974).

Corynebacterium parvum (CP). This is another microbial preparation which has received much attention. It has the considerable advantage that it is employed as a killed vaccine and is therefore devoid of the infective complica-tion of live BCG.

C. parvum is a member of the group of anaerobic corynbacteria, all pathogenic members of which have been shown to stimulate the reticulo-endothelial system. Although *C. parvum* is the organism which has been most extensively studied it is less active than other members of the group, such as *C. granulosum* and *C. anaerobium.* In fact the preparation produced by the Wellcome organisation is *C. parvum* while that produced in France by Institut Merieux is *C. avidum.*

C. parvum has been found to have a remarkable range of effects in experimental animals (see various articles in Halpern, 1975) including the stimulation of macrophages to increased phagocytosis chemotaxis and enhanced killing of ingested bacteria and of tumour cells. There is less agreement on the effect of CP on lymphocytes but some reports describe the stimulation of T and B lymphocytes, an increase in antibody synthesis against T dependent and T independent antigens, increased delayed hypersen-sitivity and lymphocytotoxicity, including lymphocytotoxicity against tumour cells. *C. parvum* has also important stimulatory activities on precursors of macrophages and lymphocytes, which suggests that CP therapy may be a useful adjunct to radiotherapy and chemotherapy which cause severe marrow depression.

C. parvum has been shown to have tumour inhibitory activities against a wide range of animal tumours (Halpern *et al.,* 1966; Woodruff and Boak, 1966; Lamensans *et al.,* 1968; Currie and Bagshawe, 1970; Smith and Scott, 1972; Israel and Halpern, 1972; Woodruff and Dunbar, 1973). The observed effects have, however, varied widely depending on the tumour examined, the size of the tumour inoculum, the route of administration of CP and the time between tumour inoculation and the administration of CP.

Many trials of *Corynebacterium parvum* in human malignant disease are in progress but their results are not yet available. Israel (in Halpern, 1975) has the most extensive experience of CP in man, having given the agent to more than four hundred patients with a wide range of malignancies. Randomised trials have been conducted in breast cancer and lung cancer, comparing the effects of chemotherapy with and without CP. The results indicate a better survival for patients receiving chemotherapy and CP and such patients suffer less from the effects of myelosuppression. Israel has also recorded synergism between CP and BCG and tumour regression after intralesional injection of CP. Early studies with CP given to patients with melanoma, acute leukaemia, sarcoma and lymphoma (Reed *et al.,* 1975) bronchogenic carcinoma (Woodruff *et al.,* 1975) and cancer of the ear, nose and throat region (Mathé, 1975) have been inconclusive. Time alone will permit evaluation of the role of *C. parvum* in oncology. For the present, it is clear that the experience of receiving CP is often an unpleasant one for the recipient (see section on complications of immunotherapy) and this has probably inhibited many physicians from using CP, with a consequent delay in its evaluation. The problem may be overcome, if the active principle of *C. parvum* can be extracted and identified and studies to this end are in progress.

Levamisole. Levamisole is an antihelminthic marketed by Janssen Pharmaceuticals, Beerse, Belgium. It has been investigated in animals and found to have effects on the functions of lymphocytes and macrophages, restoring these to normal levels where they are initially depressed (*immune restoration*) but not, apparently, inducing supranormal activity in normally functioning cells.

Studies of the effect of Levamisole on spontaneous and transplantable tumours of animals have yielded somewhat conflicting results. A majority of authors have found Levamisole to have no effect on such tumours (Chirigos *et al.,* 1973; Fidler and Spitler, 1975; Hooper *et al.,* 1975; Johnson *et al.,* 1975), but some have reported inhibition of tumour growth (Sadowski and Rapp, 1975; Takakura, 1975) and others enhanced tumour growth (Fidler and Spitler, 1975; Mantovani and Spreafico, 1975). Despite this disappointing record in animal models, attempts have been made, on the basis of its recorded ability, to increase humoral and cellular immunity including anti-tumour immunity (Shibata *et al.,* 1975; Holmes and Golub,

1976) and restore skin hypersensitivity (Brugmans *et al.*, 1973; Hirshaut *et al.*, 1977; Tripodi *et al.*, 1973) to use CP in human cancer.

In early clinical studies Levamisole was found to have *no* effect on *advanced* cancer (Ward, 1976; Symoens, 1976). Two recent reports have however suggested that Levamisole may stabilise less extended bronchogenic cancer (Amery, 1975) and breast cancer (Rojas *et al.*, 1976) and reduce the incidence of subsequent metastases.

The drug which has been relatively widely used in attempted immune restoration in non malignant conditions such as rheumatoid arthritis and aphthous oral ulceration is known to cause skin rashes and granulopaenia which may proceed to agranulocytosis. Continued cautious evaluation of Levamisole in the management of cancer seems desirable, but frequent assessment of recipients for haematological and other problems is clearly mandatory.

Many of the problems of biologically derived immunological stimulants may be largely overcome by the development of synthetic agents. The infectivity associated with living organisms would be totally abolished and the chance of anaphylactic reactions substantially reduced or abolished. It may be possible to produce agents which can selectively stimulate cellular immunity, humoral immunity or macrophage functions, depending upon which function requires to be strengthened at any given stage of disease.

Other adjuvants. As BCG, *C. parvum* and Levamisole seem unlikely to be the ideal immunostimulants there is considerable activity in searching for more effective alternative materials extracted from other organisms or artificially synthesised.

Anti-tumour properties were claimed for yeast extracts by De Backer as long ago as 1897. Supplementation of the diet with yeast (Maisin *et al.*, 1938) or yeast and B group vitamins (Lewisohn *et al.*, 1941) reduced the incidence of cancer in mice, and subsequently yeast extracts such as zymosan, hydroglucan or mannozym have been claimed to have tumour inhibiting properties (Bradner *et al.*, 1958; Diller *et al.*, 1963; Nagy *et al.*, 1971) and to increase the therapeutic effectiveness of surgery or chemotherapy in experimental murine breast carcinoma (Martin *et al.*, 1964). Maeda comprehensively reviewed the anti-tumour activity of polysaccharides in 1971 and the interested reader is recommended to consult that article. A whole host of other materials has been investigated to varying degrees and their diversity highlights the considerable, if largely unrewarded ingenuity of those interested in reticuloendothelial stimulation. For example, in the 1973 Ciba Symposium on immunopotentiation the agents discussed included *B pertussis* (Dresser), extracts of the Japanese mushroom (Dresser, Chihara), Silica and beryllium (Allison), graft versus host reactions (Katz), lymphokines (Allison), low dose of anti-lymphocyte serum (Dresser), gonadal ablation (Castro), DNCB (Hamilton) influenza virus (Lindemann) and synthetic substances such as poly IC (Woodruff). This astonishing list could be considerably expanded, but even in its present form indicates the massive task of evaluation needed to confirm or refute the utility of the substances and manipulations in it against tumours. Again the urgent requirement is for good animal models with tumour cell kinetics and antigenicity akin to human cancer.

Active specific immunotherapy

The use of general immunostimulants, regardless of their potency, is very much a hit or miss affair and there is no reason to imagine that specific anti-tumour immunity will be selectively boosted by such an approach. This is the justification for those who seek specifically to strengthen existing anti-tumour immune responses or to induce new anti-tumour responses by exposing the patient to autologous or allogeneic tumour cells or extracts of such cells, with or without concurrent administration of general immune stimulants.

It may seem illogical to take tumour cells from a patient who already bears a large volume of tumour, manipulate these cells in an arbitrary fashion, return them to the patient and hope for some specific response. It is reasonable to ask why, if the cells of a spontaneous tumour do not induce a significant tumour inhibitory immune response the administration of a relatively small number of the same tumour cells may be expected to produce this result. The evidence is, however, that this apparently bizarre procedure can alter the indices of immunity and may have clinical effects. The administration of autologous irradiated melanoma cells to patients who are anergic with respect to detectable antitumour immunity induces anti-melanoma antibodies (Ikonopisov *et al.*, 1970) and lymphocytes cytotoxic to melanoma cells (Currie *et al.*, 1971). These responses are transient but can be prolonged by combining the antigenic material with BCG (Currie *et al.*, 1971). Various explanations have been advanced to explain this curious situation. Tumour cells growing *in vivo* seem poorly immunogenic, perhaps due to the presence of masking substances manufactured by the tumour cell or blocking factors such as tumour antigens, non-cytotoxic antibody, or antigen-antibody complexes. The manipulations involved in preparing tumour cell suspensions, mechanical dispersion, enzyme treatment, minor variations in the pH of suspending and washing fluids and the process of washing by centrifugation may remove these substances or otherwise expose antigens hidden on cells growing *in vivo* and render the cells immunogenic. The phenomenon of concomitant immunity (Bashford *et al.*, 1908; Klein *et al.*, 1966) has also to be considered. This is the observation that while spontaneous tumours grow apparently unhindered *in vivo*, cells prepared from them and implanted in fresh sites in the *same animal* are rejected unless a very large challenge dose is employed. Active specific immunotherapy with autologous tumour cells probably depends upon mechanisms similar to those of concomitant immunity. Another possibility is that tumour cells produce or have associated with them materials which can selectively impede immune reactions. It has been shown that tumour cells produce materials which depress macrophage functions and extraction of tumour cell membranes, as well as yielding materials which induce delayed type cutaneous hypersensitivity reactions in cancer patients, produces materials which specifically suppress skin reactions to tumour antigens (Chapter 4). Such materials may inhibit or diminish the extent of development of immune reaction to tumour cells *in vivo*. Tumour extracts employed in immunotherapy may have no effect or an effect opposite to that intended if they are impure and contain suppressors, which may explain some previously unsuccessful trials of active specific immunotherapy. In a preliminary trial of active specific immunotherapy using highly purified extracts of bronchogenic carcinoma cell membranes, in which active and suppressive components were separated by polyacrilamide gel electrophoresis, Hollinshead and her colleagues found extended survival in recipients of this highly purified vaccine (Hollinshead and Stewart, 1977).

There are in fact numerous reports of attempts at active specific immunotherapy in man (Witebsky *et al.*, 1956; Graham and Graham, 1959; Finney *et al.*, 1960; Anderson *et al.*, 1970; March *et al.*, 1972; Ikonopisov, 1972; Southam *et al.*, 1973; Morton *et al.*, 1974: McCarthy *et al.*, 1973; Grant *et al.*, 1974; McIllmurray *et al.*, 1977). Therapists have displayed considerable ingenuity employing intact and disrupted or .extracted autologous or allogeneic tumour cells, cells treated enzymatically to remove masking coats and expose antigens (Watkins *et al.*, 1971; Simmons and Rios, 1971) and cells coupled to highly antigenic foreign proteins (Czajkowski *et al.*, 1967). Unfortunately most trials have involved relatively small numbers of patients and have been neither randomised nor concurrently controlled. The results of most reports have been similarly discouraging. However while the vast majority of patients derived no benefit from the treatment, a few had temporary remission of tumours or a pause in tumour progression. While the occurrence of even a few objective clinically detectable responses might be regarded as promising, few of the studies were designed in such a manner that one could be certain that the observed effects were not simply natural vagaries of this protean disease.

The situation is slightly more encouraging in the leukaemias with claims that combined active specific and active non-specific immunotherapy may benefit patients with acute lymphoblastic leukaemia (Mathé *et al.*, 1969, 1972), acute myeloid leukaemia (Crowther *et al.*, 1973) and chronic myeloid leukaemia (Sokal *et al.*, 1973). Active specific immunotherapy has also been successfully employed in choriocarcinoma (Bagshawe and Golding, 1971; Doniach *et al.*, 1958) but this tumour is of course a special case.

On the basis of extensive studies of immunisation in animals and man, and in particular in the light of experience of the induction of experimental organ-specific autoimmune disease, the optimum method of producing anti-tumour immunity *should* be the injection of tumour antigens with an adjuvant. That this has not so far been highly successful is frustrating but may merely reflect the impurity of the antigenic preparations employed and the presence of inhibitors. If this problem can be overcome we will hear much more of active specific immunotherapy. If naturally occurring tumour associated antigens lack the capacity to induce rejection producing reactions, and we cannot modify them to develop this desirable characteristic, alternative approaches will need to be sought.

Local immunotherapy

In contrast to the systemic administration of immunological adjuvants outlined above, there is considerable interest in the application of adjuvant materials directly to accessible tumours. This involves the injection of materials into the tumour substance or the application of contact-sensitisors to the tissues overlying the tumour. A considerable range of agents has been investigated including BCG (Morton *et al.*, 1970; Nathanson, 1972; Pinsky *et al.*, 1972; Grant *et al.*, 1974; Serrou *et al.*, 1975; Zbar *et al.*, 1975) dinitro-chlorobenzene (Klein, 1969; Stjernswärd and Levin, 1971; Malek-Mansour

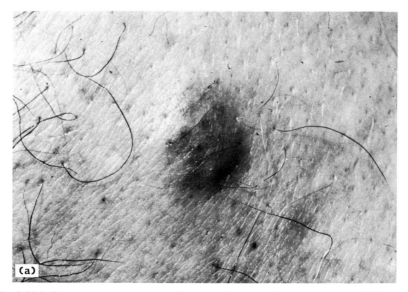

Fig. 8.2(a). Cutaneous secondary malignant melanoma prior to intralesional injection of BCG.

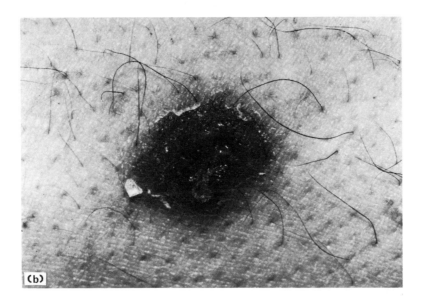

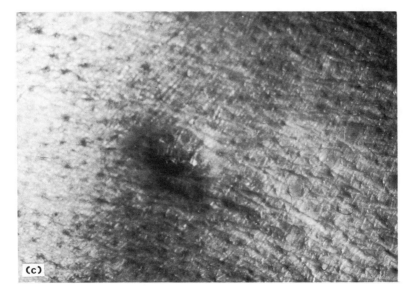

Fig. 8.2 (cont.)

(b). Cutaneous secondary malignant melanoma showing ulceration, two weeks after intralesional injection of BCG.

(c). Cutaneous secondary malignant melanoma showing total resolution ten weeks after intralesional injection of BCG.

et al., 1973), vaccinia virus (Burdick, 1960; Belisario and Milton, 1961; Milton and Lane Brown, 1966; Dent *et al.*, 1972; Everall *et al.*, 1975), *Corynebacterium parvum* (Israel *et al.*, 1975), varidase (Stewart and Tolnai, 1969), *in vitro* activated autochthonous lymphocytes (Cheema and Hersh, 1972) and fractions of the serum of patients who had been immunised with autologous tumour cells and Freund's adjuvant (Finney *et al.*, 1960).

The findings have been basically similar regardless of the agent applied. A delayed hypersensitivity reaction develops in and around the treated area (Fig. 8.2a), ulceration follows (Fig. 8.2b) and the lesion then heals leaving a depressed scar (Fig. 8.2c). Microscopy shows the tumour infiltrated by lymphocytes and macrophages (Fig. 8.3), sometimes with poorly formed giant cell containing follicular granulomas in the case of BCG (Fig. 8.4). The tumour cells are seen in various stages of necrosis and disintegration (Fig. 8.3). Resolution of the tumour is usually complete in 4 to 6 weeks.

There is considerable debate as to whether this dramatic effect is a purely local one or whether a degree of systemic response occurs. Morton *et al.*, (1974) found that 16% of non-injected tumours regressed. Our own

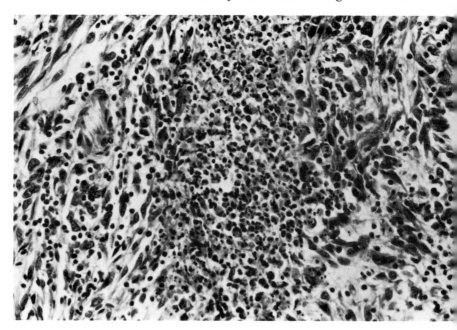

Fig. 8.3. Photomicrograph of a cutaneous secondary malignant melanoma two weeks after intralesional injection of BCG. The tumour is infiltrated by lymphocytes and macrophages and the tumour cells show varying stages of necrosis and disintegration. Haematoxylin and Eosin (× 250).

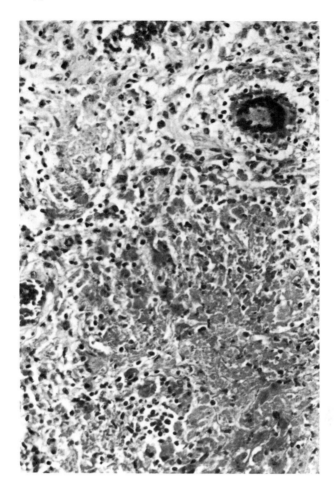

Fig. 8.4. Photomicrograph of a cutaneous secondary malignant melanoma two weeks after intralesional injectionof BCG showing Langhans-type giant cell formation. Haematoxylin and Eosin (× 250).

experience with this technique confirms that a minority of non-injected nodules do regress, but we have observed uninjected nodules less than 10 mm. from injected regressing nodules to be unaffected (Fig. 8.5). Where we have encountered regression of non-injected nodules they have usually lain within the same lymphatic drainage area as injected nodules, often between the injected nodule and the nearest draining lymph node. That BCG mycobacteria are disseminated after intratumoral injection is proved by the occurrence of mycobacteria containing granulomata in the liver and other organs of patients treated in this way and Mathé regards this dissemination

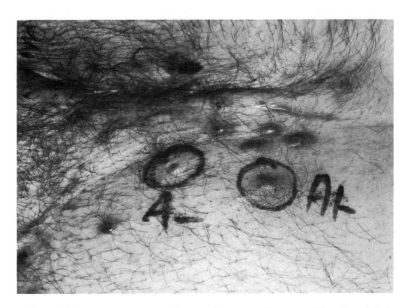

Fig. 8.5. Multiple cutaneous secondary malignant melanomas. The ringed lesion on the right (A+) shows a delayed hypersensitivity response following intralesional injection of BCG. The closely adjacent ringed lesion on the left (A—) received no BCG and shows no alteration.

as a critical element in BCG treatment (see above). Alterations in tumour-directed antibodies and lymphocytes do occur in patients receiving BCG, even in those with disseminated disease, indicating a systemic effect of BCG (Cochran *et al.*, 1978). That the systemic effect is not very strong is indicated by the progression of visceral metastases despite local control of accessible cutaneous or mucosal lesions by local immunotherapy. However it is probable that the number of tumour involved in visceral metastases is grossly in excess of that which may be controlled by anti-tumour immunity.

While it may seem pointless to control minor non life-threatening cutaneous deposits in the face of lethal visceral metastases, there are excellent humanitarian reasons for undertaking local therapy. Patients are often very distressed by visible tumour deposits which continually remind them of the seriousness of their condition. By contrast they are often unaware of, or able to suppress concern about invisible visceral tumour deposits which will eventually kill them. We recently had a patient who was very distressed by carcinomatous recurrences on her mastectomy scar (Fig. 8.6a) and embarrassed by their breakdown and the offensive odour from a continuous purulent discharge. The lesions resolved promptly after intra-lesional BCG and the wound healed (Fig. 8.6b). Her disease progressed

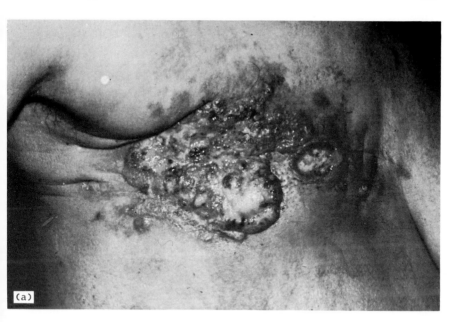

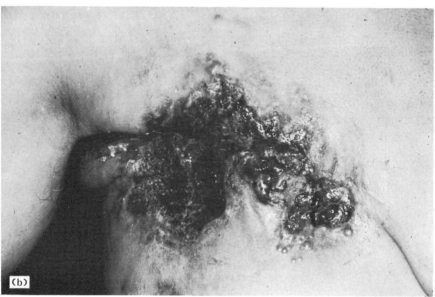

Fig. 8.6(a). Local recurrences of breast carcinoma in the area of a mastectomy scar prior to intralesional injection of BCG.
(b). Resolution of lesions depicted in Figure 8.6a six weeks after intralesional injection of BCG. (Photographs by courtesy of Dr. R. M. Grant.)

during the subsequent year, with continued development of visceral metastases but the absence of visible tumour made it easier for her to make appropriate psychological adjustments to her situation. It may be argued that accessible lesions are just as effectively treated by surgical removal or radiotherapy. However the administration of intralesional immunotherapy can readily be managed on an outpatient basis and allows the patient to spend more time at home. This type of approach has also much to commend it in the elderly where repeated general anaesthesia or hospitalisation are especially undesirable.

These techniques have until recently, been employed mainly in the treatment of intradermal metastases and most authors have had little success with deeper seated lesions. There are now reports of the use of DNCB and intralesional therapy in the treatment of primary tumours. The aim in most studies has been to treat the primary melanoma prior to surgical excision (e.g. Everall *et al.*, 1975) but Malek-Mansour and her collaborators (1973), on the basis of a low incidence of metastases in patients whose primaries were treated with DNCB followed by surgery, have recently initiated a trial of DNCB sensitisation and challenge as the sole therapy for primary malignant melanoma (Malek-Mansour, personal communication). The local treatment of tumours in this way is widely applicable, can be used to treat multiple lesions on one patient and with a little ingenuity can be applied to tumours arising in non-cutaneous sites such as the vagina, uterine cervix and bladder. It is not, however, without hazard (see below) and patients treated in this way require especially frequent and close surveillance.

The mechanism of tumour destruction by local immunotherapy is incompletely understood. The consensus until recently was that the tumour was destroyed in a non-specific fashion by the cells involved in the induced delayed hypersensitivity reaction to the immunising agent; the tumour in the very limited context of this argument being an innocent bystander. It has recently been suggested (Zbar and Rapp, 1974) that while the initial reaction to local immunotherapy is not tumour specific, there may develop, after the initial breakdown of tumour cells with release of tumour antigens, a degree of enhanced specific immunity to complement the initial non-specific effects. This interesting suggestion remains unproven.

PASSIVE IMMUNOTHERAPY

Passive immunotherapy with anti-tumour antibodies

This approach has much to commend it on theoretical grounds. The exquisite specificity of immunoglobulin combining sites will direct appropriate antibodies to tumour associated antigens and if the antibodies can bind complement or sensitise tumour cells for K cell attack, will bring about the destruction of cells bearing the requisite antigens. Enthusiasm has, of course to be tempered by the possibility of antibody-mediated blocking. If anti-tumour antibodies and lymphocytes are not induced spontaneously or are incapable of exerting a controlling influence on tumour cells and we lack the knowledge to induce or appropriately magnify an anti-tumour response one possible answer is to use antibodies or lymphocytes raised against tumour associated antigens in other members of the same species or in members of other species. Some encouragement for this latter approach is provided by nature. There are reports of tumour regression following the administration of sera from patients with cured or spontaneously regressing tumours (Sumner and Foraker, 1960; Teimourian and McCune, 1963; Ngu, 1967; Nathanson et al., 1967; Horn and Horn, 1971). Unfortunately this seems an exceptional situation and there are many reports of unsuccessful attempts at serotherapy (Southam, 1961; Harris and Sinkovics, 1970; Order et al., 1974) and one suspects a considerable number of unreported failures. The reasons for the success or failure of allogeneic serotherapy are quite unknown, and this seems a worthwhile and accessible area of study. The availability of a suitable serum donor may present problems, but there are reports of attempts to raise anti-tumour serum and lymphocytes by inoculating tumour from one individual into another (Nadler and Moore, 1965; Willoughby et al., 1970; Marsh et al., 1972). Those considering this approach should, however, be aware of the potential hazards of this procedure; there being reports of tumour progression in and death of tumour allograft recipients (e.g. Scanlon et al., 1965).

Logistic and ethical problems involved in the provision of allogeneic anti-tumour sera have led to investigations of the possibility of employing xenogeneic antisera. Tumour antigens are generally "weak" by comparison with species, transplantation and organ specific antigens and until recently it has not been possible to obtain purified tumour antigens for immunisation purposes. It has therefore been necessary to absorb xenogeneic anti-sera with normal tissues of different kinds to render them tumour-specific and there has often been doubt as to whether weak anti-tumour activity would survive this treatment. Pressman et al. (1953, 1958) studied this problem extensively and showed that labelled antibodies to experimental animal tumours do retain the ability to localise in the tumours even after extensive absorptions. These findings cannot of course be extrapolated beyond the specific experiments described and all xenogeneic antisera need to be carefully assessed for residual anti-tumour activity after absorption.

The use of foreign serum carries the dangers of anaphylaxis, serum sickness and glomerular damage from foreign protein-host antibody complexes and problems of this kind have been encountered in studies employing these sera. Current understanding of the mechanisms of these undesirable effects should permit a substantial reduction in the risk of their occurrence making the use of foreign sera a more acceptable proposition.

Having raised a xenogeneic anti-tumour antiserum, absorbed out all activity against normal tissue components and modified it to minimise the occurrence of undesirable side effects, the serum, while capable of reacting with tumour antigens *in vivo* may lack the capacity to kill tumour cells. An ingenious possibility, is to use the specificity of the impotent antibodies to carry cytotoxic reagents to the tumour cells and in this way achieve a locally cytotoxic level of drug. Mathé *et al.* (1958) diazotised methotrexate to a mouse antileukaemia serum and found it to be more effective than either the serum or drug alone in protecting leukaemia challenged animals. Ghose *et al.* (1972a and b) found that xenoantibodies to the tumour antigens of the murine lymphoma EL4 and the Ehrlich ascites tumour, could substantially inhibit tumour growth when associated with chlorambucil. They attempted to apply this approach to patients with melanoma and recorded one striking success (Ghose *et al.*, 1972b). Other workers attracted by this promising approach, have found that the antibody-chlorambucil association is loose and probably non-covalent, and that drug and antibody rapidly dissociate when introduced *in vivo*. Studies are therefore in progress to devise means whereby chlorambucil and antibody or other cytotoxic drugs and antibody may be covalently linked without substantially destroying the antigenic specificity of the immunoglobulin molecule. In the meantime Davies and O'Neil (1973) report that covalent linkage of antibody and drug or linkage of any kind may be unnecessary and that the administration of chlorambucil followed by anti-tumour antibody achieves a therapeutic effect considerably in excess of either alone. Drug given after the antibody does not show enhanced tumour cell killing. The authors conclude that antibody can kill drug affected tumour cells, but antibody affected cells are not specially sensitive to the drug.

Adoptive immunotherapy with lymphocytes

It might seem curious to consider the employment of the patients' own lymphocytes when these have failed to control the tumour spontaneously *in vivo*. Such an approach is worth consideration only if the performance of autologous lymphocytes can be improved. This may be possible by the removal of lymphocytes and their education *in vitro* (Hardy *et al.*, 1970; Golub *et al.*, 1972). Lymphocytes which after exposure to tumour cells *in vitro* acquire the ability to kill target cells bearing the same membrane antigens as the stimulating cells may provide a valuable therapeutic tool. Activation of lymphocytes *in vitro* by mitogens is a technically simpler, though non-specific alternative. As most *in vitro* studies suggest that many lymphocytes are needed to kill a tumour cell this approach is likely to succeed only if the population of sensitised lymphocytes can be magnified by, for instance large scale culture *in vitro*. It would also seem desirable to present the tumour antigens in as highly immunogenic a form as possible and antigenic "improvement" of tumour cells by enzymatic removal of masking coats may be a necessary part of *"in vitro"* education.

Lymphocytes from sources other than the patient can be used to provide either specifically sensitised cells or non-sensitised cells (Woodruff and Nolan, 1963). The latter, while readily available, seem unlikely to survive sufficiently long in the recipient to undergo *in vivo* education and in any case, the recognition of and reaction to tumour specific antigen would seem likely to be only part, and probably not a very major part, of a complex reaction to species, strain and organ markers. Sensitised lymphocytes from allogeneic donors may be obtained from patients who have responded to therapy or whose tumours have undergone spontaneous regression or from family members or laboratory personnel who may have shown "spontaneous" sensitisation to the relevant TAA perhaps by exposure to the same carcinogens as the patient (Chapter 3) (Yonemoto and Terasaki, 1972).

It is also possible to induce sensitization of the lymphocytes of a normal donor by immunisation, but the dangers of this have been outlined above. Studies of immunisation for the induction of therapeutic materials have for ethical reasons often employed the exchange of tumour material between cancer patients with subsequent reverse exchange of lymphocytes and/or serum (Nadler and Moore, 1965; Andrews *et al.*, 1967; Marsh *et al.*, 1972; Oon *et al.*, 1975). The results of such experiments have not, in general, been encouraging, although a minority of patients are claimed to have had some benefit from the procedure. The main problem with allogeneic (or xenogeneic) lymphocytes is that their life in the recipient seems likely to be short as they will be recognised as foreign and rejected promptly on this basis. It is possible, however, that while the intact cells have a short existence, as they are destroyed they may bequeath important "information" to the host lymphocytes, for instance by the release of transfer factor or immune RNA (see below). It is perfectly possible to prolong the survival of such lymphocytes by inducing immunological suppression, however this carries its own problems. The grafted lymphocytes may cause a graft versus host reaction (Andrews *et al.*, 1967) and additionally, since they too will be subject to the effects of the immunosuppressive regime, their anti-tumour activity may be less than could otherwise be expected.

Attempts to induce and employ specifically sensitised xenogeneic lympho-cytes (Symes *et al.*, 1968, 1973a, b) have not been strikingly successful and the problems of selective immunisation against tumour associated antigens and rapid destruction of donor lymphocytes by the host versus graft reaction remain to be solved. Immunisation with tumour material either preceded by or followed by tolerisation to the equivalent normal tissues seems a possible way round this problem.

Immunotherapy with lymphocyte extracts and products

Transfer factor. Lawrence (1955, 1969) has shown that a fraction of low molecular weight which could be extracted from the lymphocytes of tuberculin reactive guinea pigs was able to transfer this reactivity passively to non-reactive animals. In man antigenic sensitisation can also be transferred in this way to normal recipients and to cancer patients, although the acquired reactivity is short lasting in the latter group (Rapaport and Lawrence, 1975). Transfer factor has been used, with some success in the management of immunological deficiency states (Lawrence, 1969; Levin *et al.*, 1970) and viral, fungal and mycobacterial infections where an aberration of T cell function is implicated (Lawrence, 1969). In view of the postulated immune deficiency in malignant disease, there have been attempts to use transfer factor in cancer patients (Goldenberg and Brandes, 1972; Levin *et al.*, 1975). Pilot studies have been inconclusive, but not entirely negative and alterations in lymphocyte subpopulations have followed this treatment (Levin *et al.*, 1975), encouraging the establishment of the more formal trials currently in progress.

"Immune" RNA. This material may be extracted from the lymphoid organs or peripheral blood lymphocytes of sensitised animals and can confer the ability to synthesise specific anti-phage antibodies (Fishman, 1961) and immunity against skin allografts (Mannick and Egdahl, 1964; Sabbadini and Sehon, 1967) and tumours (Ramming and Pilch, 1970; Deckers and Pilch, 1971; Deckers *et al.*, 1975). Immune RNA extracted from the lymphoid tissues of sheep and guinea pigs immunised against human tumours can induce anti-tumour cytolytic activity *in vitro* in normal human lymphocytes (Veltman *et al.*, 1974; Pilch *et al.*, 1975), as can "immune" RNA from patients "cured" of malignancy (Pilch *et al.*, 1975). The immune RNA molecule is three to four times the size of the transfer factor molecule, but its exact nature remains to be elucidated and the possibility that transfer factor is included within it cannot be excluded. Cautious preliminary attempts to employ "Immune" RNA in the therapy of human cancer are in progress (Pilch—personal communication).

Lymphocyte products. The dramatic tumour regressions seen after intralesional immunotherapy are largely due to the effects of lymphocyte activation products (lymphokines). There is considerable interest in the production of substances such as immune interferon, migration inhibition factor and lymphotoxin on a scale sufficiently large to allow investigation of the effects of their systemic administration on patients with malignant disease. Improved techniques for the culture of lymphocytes and the recognition that mitogen stimulated lymphocytes yield lymphokines make this type of investigation more practical.

Thymic extracts. The exact means whereby the thymus gland exerts its effects remain unknown. There is, however, considerable evidence that it operates by producing hormones which are most probably produced by the epithelial component. A major function of such hormones would be to commit lymphocytes to function as T cells. If such an activity were in abeyance, either as part of ageing or as a result of the activities of micro-organisms or chemicals, including drugs, T lymphocyte activities of micro-their activities against tumour cells, would be reduced. Various thymic extracts have been prepared and examined in animal systems and more recently in man. If thymic dysfunction is found to be important in oncogenesis or the progression of cancer, replacement therapy with thymic hormone would seem a logical therapeutic approach (see leader in British Medical Journal, 1977 for review).

Complications of Immunotherapy

IMMUNOTHERAPY WITH BCG

The great majority of patients who receive BCG are little incommoded by their therapy, particularly when the BCG is administered intradermally by scarification, Heaf gun or an equivalent technique. Most experience influenza-like symptoms which commence 12-24 hours after receiving the BCG and usually subside within 48 hours of their onset, although they may persist for longer in a few patients. The main symptoms are malaise, shivering, nausea and anorexia associated with a small increase in temperature. These symptoms are often sufficiently severe to prevent attendance at work or performance of domestic duties and for this reason many patients elect to have their BCG prior to the weekend.

Local problems at the site of administration of intradermal BCG are unusual although the extensive crusting, scarring and occasional depigmentation of the scratch or puncture marks are unsightly and may make the prospect of prolonged therapy unattractive, especially to young women (Fig. 8.7). The injection of BCG mixed with irradiated or formalinised tumours cells in active specific immunotherapy and intralesional BCG may be associated with the formation of abscesses which produce surprisingly large quantities of pus over a period of weeks or months (Nathanson, 1972; Pinsky et al., 1972). Live BCG organisms are readily cultured from these lesions and caution in the handling and disposal of infected dressings is

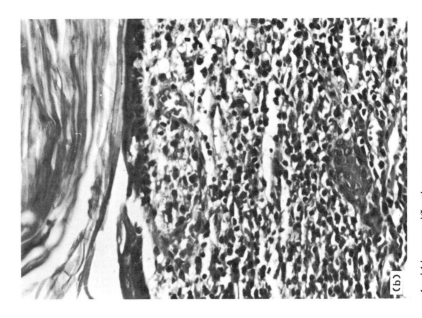

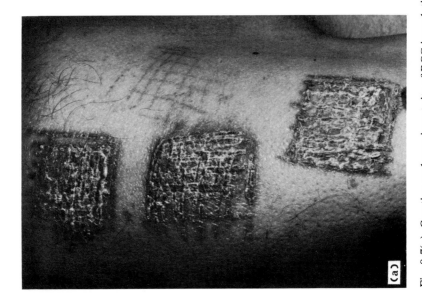

Fig. 8.7(a). Crusting and scarring at site of BCG inoculation into needle formed grid iron scarifications. (b). Photomicrograph of scarified site. Haematoxylin and Eosin (×300).

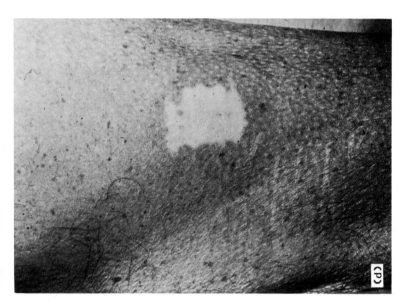

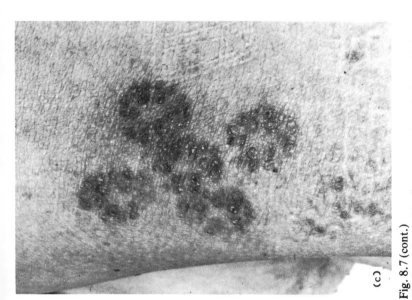

Fig. 8.7 (cont.)
(c). Scars formed by five pressure inoculations of BCG by a Heaf gun. Note adjacent depigmented scarification lines.
(d). Depigmentation of an area of scarring following grid iron inoculation of BCG.

appropriate, especially in the domestic situation. The pathogenicity of BCG to the immunologically normal individual is low, but if large numbers of patients are receiving BCG it is possible that immunodepressed individuals could inadvertently be infected from a source of this kind with potentially disastrous consequences.

Many patients who are receiving BCG develop minor degrees of liver dysfunction indicated by alterations in liver function tests, especially in the enzyme patterns. These enzyme changes respond at least partially to anti-tuberculous therapy in most patients suggesting that mycobacteria are involved in the causation of this condition. Liver biopsy examination of BCG recipients showing hepatic dysfunction has shown tuberculoid granulomata in the liver of a proportion of patients; granulomatous hepatitis (Freundlich and Suprun, 1969; Hunt et al., 1973; Sparks et al., 1973; Serrou et al., 1975). We have found lesions of this kind at autopsy in several patients dying of melanomatosis (Fig. 8.8) and have readily demonstrated mycobacteria in them by appropriate special stains. It now seems certain that a mycobacterial bacteraemia follows the administration of BCG and Mathé claims that this is a necessary and desirable event for the development of immunostimulant effects (see above). Such lesions seem likely to be persistent in the absence of anti-tuberculous therapy as Gormsen (1955) has shown that children dying of other causes some years after administration of conventionally low doses of BCG for tuberculosis prophylaxis had a few typical granulomata in the liver. In the fact of multiple foci of myocbacteria, even those of low pathogeneicity, care must be exercised if high doses of steroids or other immunodepressive drugs are administered concurrently with or subsequent to high dose BCG therapy.

Spread of the mycobacteria from the site of their introduction to the draining lymph nodes seems an inevitable concomitant of BCG administration. Mildly tender enlargement of the draining lymph nodes has occurred in a minority of our patients receiving BCG, but we have not encountered persisting lymphadenopathy or mycobacterial abscesses of the lymph nodes, although these complications have been recorded by others (Chaves-Carballo and Sanchez, 1972; Watkins, 1971).

The development of a generalised progressive infection with BCG is fortunately rare (Matsaniotis, 1967; Watanabe et al., 1969; Esterley et al., 1971) but does occur and was a major contributory cause of death in one of the first of our patients to receive BCG (Grant et al., 1974). This patient received a massive total dose of BCG, a dose which we would now regard as excessive, in divided doses over six months as intralesional injections and scarifications. He developed a chest radiographic appearance which suggested either diffuse carcinomatosis or a chronic infection (Fig. 8.9). Sputa were persistently negative for mycobacteria and his clinical response to

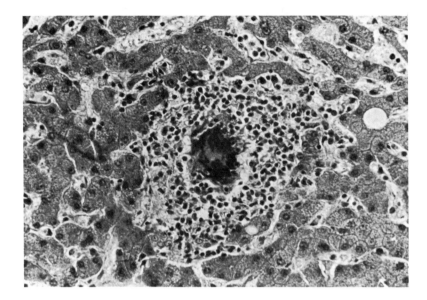

Fig. 8.8. Photomicrograph of a tuberculoid granuloma of liver in a patient receiving BCG by scarification. Haematoxylin and Eosin (× 400).

pragmatic anti-tuberculous therapy was minimal. He died of a myocardial infarction and at autopsy had an extensive mycobacterial bronchopneumonia with granulomata in the liver, kidneys, spleen and adrenal as well as the lung. This disastrous complication has also been recorded by others and may in part be a result of terminal tumour related immune depression. It has been said to be almost exclusively a sequel of intralesional BCG but we have enountered it in two patients who had received BCG only by scarification. Early detection of this condition is essential and demands frequent follow up assessment of patients at risk, with radiographic monitoring of the chest, and a high index of awareness of the possibility of its occurrence. Early deployment of anti-tuberculous therapy rapidly resolved the condition in the two patients referred to above.

Deaths have also been recorded as a result of anaphylactic reactions to BCG, with high fever and major coagulation failure, and the appropriate resuscitative materials must be available whenever BCG is to be given, although even strenuous resuscitation has not always reversed anaphylaxis in this situation (McKhann et al., 1975; Diamond, 1968). Rarer complications of BCG therapy include lichen scrofulosum (Warner, 1966), and osteomyelitis (Erikson and Hjelmstedt, 1971).

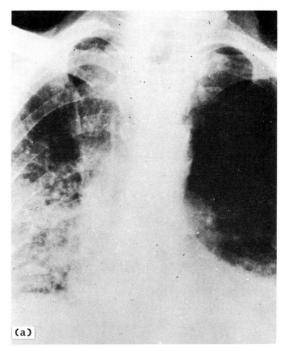

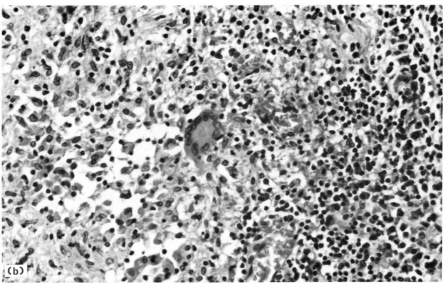

Fig. 8.9(a). Chest x-ray of patient with disseminated BCG infection. (b) At autopsy
the lungs showed a predominantly mononuclear cell pneumonia with occasional giant
cells. Mycobacteria were identified in the granulomas. Haematoxylin and Eosin
(×300).

IMMUNOTHERAPY WITH CORYNEBACTERIUM PARVUM (CP)

In man administration of CP, by whatever route, is associated with a febrile reaction which is usually of short duration and may reduce in severity with successive doses. Subcutaneous and intralesional injections cause pain which is usually tolerable but rarely may be sufficiently severe that treatment by this route must be stopped. Intratumoral injections produce major local inflammation sometimes progressing to suppuration. Intraperitoneal and intravenous injections are said to be well tolerated (Israel, 1975), although Woodruff et al. (1975) and Reed et al. (1975) found systemic reactions more pronounced in patients receiving intravenous CP, and Woodruff et al. record one case of hepatotoxicity. Mild cardiovascular changes, transient hypotension or hypertension were observed in CP recipients by Reed et al. (1975). Extended evaluation of CP in man may uncover other problems and there is currently concern that diffuse intravascular coagulation, thrombocytopaenia and nephrotic syndrome may develop in a minority of CP recipients.

IMMUNOTHERAPY WITH LEVAMISOLE

Levamisole is well tolerated by most cancer patients and the problems encountered have been, with a few significant exceptions, minor. Side effects are said to be most common in patients with rheumatoid arthritis. A few patients have developed skin rashes and high doses may be associated with gastrointestinal symptoms (Symöens, 1976). Granulopaenia has been not uncommon and recently there have been several worrying reports of agranulocytosis after Levamisole (Graber et al., 1976; Rosenthal et al., 1976; Ruuskanen et al., 1976; Williams, 1976; Van Holder and Van Hove, 1977). The requirement for close haematological assessment of all patients on this drug is clear.

ACTIVE SPECIFIC IMMUNOTHERAPY

No major problems have yet been observed which relate to the administration of tumour cell or tumour cell extracts. The potential growth of living allogeneic tumour cells in immunosuppressed recipients dictates that such cells be rendered incapable of replication by irradiation or chemical treatment prior to their administration. The use of allogeneic tumour cells carries the theoretical risk of introducing oncogenic viruses or oncogenes and this possibility cannot at present be excluded. It would probably require time for such agents to cause trouble and the sad fact is that very few patients treated with allogeneic tumour cells survive their existing carcinoma for any substantial length of time.

PASSIVE IMMUNOTHERAPY

The main problems here are anaphylaxis, serum sickness and glomerulonephritis after the administration of allogeneic or xenogeneic serum and graft versus host disease when foreign immunocompetent cells are given. There is insufficient experience of the other forms of passive immunotherapy to allow any firm statement on problems associated with their use.

The dreaded complication of tumour enhancement has been recorded sporadically in a small minority of patients receiving a variety of forms of immunotherapy. It is, however, difficult to see how this may be identified in an inherently variable disease other than within the framework of a prospective, randomised concurrently controlled trial. In this context the recent report of melanoma enhancement by active specific immunotherapy from McIllmurray et al. (1977) is worrying. However, the trial was abandoned at an early stage and while one sympathises with the appalling ethical dilemma of the physicians conducting this trial, the small number of patients observed makes the conclusions drawn unconvincing.

Monitoring of Patients Receiving Immunotherapy

The general considerations discussed in the section on immunological monitoring of cancer patients (Chapter 6) apply equally to the recipients of immunotherapy. Serial studies of the immunology of immunotherapy patients are in progress in many centres (Gutterman et al., 1973; Cohen et al., 1974; McGrath, 1975; Serrou et al., 1975; Golub et al., 1976) and it seems that detectable variations in immune reactions parallel tumour regression and progression and may under certain circumstances predict tumour recurrence and metastasis formation. I have previously outlined our own approach to this activity (Chapter 6). Our present results obtained from the immunological monitoring of patients receiving immunotherapy suggest that our tests reflect medium term variations in tumour growth rather than short term alterations induced by immunotherapy (Mackie et al., In Press). The results of our own studies (Cochran et al., 1977) and those of others are encouraging but the techniques remain cumbersome and the results insufficiently clear to permit the routine clinical use of currently available monitoring systems. Monitoring by serial estimations of tumour markers such as CEA and HCG is certainly applicable to immunotherapy patients, but is unfortunately limited to only a few tumours at present.

Tests are available to measure the specific response to immunotherapeutic agents such as BCG in vivo and in vitro and indicate that a majority of patients do develop or strengthen an immune reaction to the agent employed (Cochran et al., 1977). It is by no means certain, however, that a good response of this kind necessarily predicts a good clinical response.

Monitoring of immunotherapy patients must therefore depend for the present largely upon the established methods of clinical examination supplemented where appropriate by radiology, scintigraphy, ultrasonography and biochemistry. A knowledge of the complications likely with each agent permits selective examinations to be undertaken; BCG recipients, for instance, requiring close scrutiny of their liver enzymes to detect granulomatous hepatitis and repeated chest radiography to exclude disseminated "BCGosis".

Summary

One cannot fail to be impressed by the ingenuity manifest in the veritable cornucopia of approaches to immunotherapy. There is little doubt that a few of the current techniques will find a place in the treatment of cancer, even if only for a short time and until superseded by better techniques and materials. Evaluation is a major task since men are not like the conveniently short lived laboratory animals and their living and dying occupies many years rather than weeks or months. Unreasonable expectations and a desire for instant results (and gratifications) have led to disappointment with immunotherapy and it would be unfortunate if this were to develop into an emotional climate which hampered its continued careful evaluation. There is no evidence that immunotherapy is likely, in the foreseeable future, to develop as a sole treatment for cancer and it would be highly undesirable if these new techniques were considered as in any sense competitive with the existing forms of treatment. The existing evidence points to immunotherapy as merely one weapon in the therapeutic armoury and our business is *simply* to identify those (perhaps few) situations in which it can most appropriately and effectively be employed. While this information will be partly available from clinical trial and error there is a continuing requirement for clinical immunologists involved in this area to scrutinise the advancing knowledge of basic immunology for relevant observations and techniques. Those who award research funds, and who are currently enthusiastic for "goal-oriented" research, would do well to take this into consideration.

References

Adam, A., Ciorbanu, R., Petit, J. F. and Lederer, E. (1972). *Proc. nat. Acad. Sci. USA* **69**, 851.

Amery, W. (1975). *Brit. med. J.* **3**, 461.

Anderson, J. M., deSousa, M. A. B., Halnan, K. E., Kelly, F. and Hannah, G. (1970). *Brit. J. Surg.* **57**, 557.

Andrews, G. A., Congdon, C. C., Edwards, C. L., Gengozian, N., Nelson, B. and Vodopick, H. (1967). *Cancer Res.* **27**, 2535.

Aur, R., Verzosa, M., Hustu, O., Simone, J. and Barker, L. (1975). *Proc. Amer. Assoc. Cancer Res.* **16**, 92 (Abstract).

Bagshawe, K. D. and Golding, P. R. (1971). "Immunity and Tolerance in Oncogenesis." University of Perugia, Perugia, Italy.

Baldwin, R. W. and Pimm, M. V. (1973). *Int. J. Cancer* **28**, 282.

Balner, H., Old, L. J. and Clarke, D. A. (1962). *Proc. Soc. exp. Biol. Med.* **109**, 58.

Bashford, E. F., Murray, J. A., Haaland, M. and Bowen, W. H. (1908). *Third Sci. Rep. Imp. Cancer Res. Fund (London)* **3**, 262.

Belisario, J. C. and Milton, G. W. (1961). *Aust. J. Dermatol.* **6**, 113.

Biozzi, G., Benacerraf, B., Grunback, F., Halpern, B. N., Levadite, J. and Rist, N. (1954). *Ann. Inst. Pasteur Lille* **87**, 291.

Biozzi, G., Stiffel, C., Halpern, B. N. and Mouton, D. (1959). *C.R. Soc. Biol. (Paris)* **153**, 987.

Bluming, A. Z., Vogel, C. L., Ziegler, J. L., Mody, N., Kamya, G. and Uganda, K. (1972). *Ann. intern. Med.* **76**, 405.

Bradner, W. T., Clarke, D. A. and Stock, C. C. (1958). *Cancer Res.* **18**, 347.

Brody, J. A. and McAlister, R. (1964). *Am. Rev. resp. Dis.* **90**, 607.

Brugmans, J., Schuermans, V., deCock, W., Thienpunt, D., Janssen, P., Verhaegen, H., van Nimmen, L., Louwagie, A. C. and Stevens, E. (1973). *Life Sciences* **13**, 1499.

Burchenal, J. H. (1966). *Cancer Res.* **26**, 2393.

Burdick, K. H. (1960). *Arch. Derm.* **82**, 438.

Carter, S. K. and Slavik, M. (1975). *In* "Corynebacterium parvum" (B. Halpern, Ed.) 329. Plenum Press, New York.

Chaves-Carballo, E. and Sanchez, G. A. (1972). *Clin. Pediatr. (Philad.)* **11**, 693.

Cheema, A. R. and Hersh, E. M. (1972). *Cancer* **29**, 982.

Chirigos, M. A., Pearson, J. W. and Pryor, J. (1973). *Cancer Res.* **33**, 2615.

Cleveland, R., Meltzer, M. S. and Zbar, B. (1974). *J. nat. Cancer Inst.* **52**, 1887.

Cochran, A. J. (1969). *Cancer* **23**, 1190.

Cochran, A. J., Mackie, R. M., Jackson, A. M., Ogg, L. J. and Ross, C. E. (1978). *Dev. Biol. Stand.* **38**, 441.

Cohen, M. H., Chretien, P. B., Felix, E. L., Lloyd, B. C., Ketcham, A. S., Albright, L. A. and Ommaya, A. K. (1974). *Nature* **249**, 656.

Coley, W. B. (1891). *Ann. Surg.* **14**, 199.

Coley, W. B. (1893). *Med. Rec.* **43**, 60.

Comstock, G. W., Livesay, V. T. and Webster, R. G. (1971). *Lancet* **2**, 1062.

Comstock, G. W., Martinez, I. and Livesay, V. T. (1975). *J. nat. Cancer Inst.* **54**, 835.

Crowther, D., Powles, R., Bateman, C. J. T., Beard, M. E. J., Gauci, C. L., Wrigley, P. F. M., Malpas, J. S., Hamilton Fairley, G. and Bodley, S. R. (1973). *Brit. med. J.* **1**, 131.

Currie, G. A. and Bagshawe, K. D. (1970). *Brit. med. J.* **1**, 541.

Currie, G. A., Lejeune, F. and Fairley, G. H. (1971). *Brit. med. J.* **2**, 305.

Czajkowski, N. D., Rosenblatt, M., Wolf, P. L. and Vasquez, J. (1967). *Lancet* **2**, 905.

Davies, D. A. L. and O'Neill, G. J. (1973). *Brit. J. Cancer* **28**, Suppl. 1, 285.

Davignon, L., Lemonde, P., Robillard, P. and Frappier, A. (1970). *Lancet* **2**, 638.

deBacker, J. (1897). *J. Méd. de Paris* **2**, 276.

Deckers, P. J. and Pilch, Y. H. (1971). *Cancer* **28**, 1219.

Deckers, P. J., Wang, B. S., Stuart, P. A. and Mannick, J. A. (1975). *In* "Cancer and Transplantation" (Murphy, G. P., Ed.) Grune and Stratton, New York.

Dent, R. I., Cruickshank, J. G., Gordon, J. A. and Swanepole, R. (1972). *C. Afr. J. Med.* **18**, 173.

Diamond, J. (1968). *Lancet* **2**, 875.

Dienes, L. (1936). *Arch. Pathol.* **21**, 357.

Diller, I. C., Mankowski, Z. T. and Fisher, M. E. (1963). *Cancer Res.* **23**, 201.

Doniach, I., Crookston, J. H. and Cope, T. I. (1958). *J. Obstet. Gynaec. Br. Emp.* **65,** 553.

Dubois, R. J. and Schaedler, R. W. (1957). *J. exp. Med.* **106,** 703.

EORTC Haemopathies Working Party (1975). *Proc. Third Meeting Internat. Soc. Haemotol. (Europe and African Div.),* London.

Erikson, U. and Hjelmstedt, A. (1971). *Radiology* **101,** 575.

Esterly, J. R., Sturner, W. Q., Esterly, N. B. and Windhorst, D. B. (1971). *Pediatrics* **48,** 141.

Evans, R. and Alexander, P. (1972). *Nature* **236,** 168.

Everall, J. D., O'Doherty, C. J., Wand, J. and Dowd, P. M. (1975). *Lancet* **2,** 583.

Fidler, I. J. and Spitler, L. E. (1975). *J. nat. Cancer Inst.* **55,** 1107.

Finney, J. W., Byers, E. H. and Wilson, R. H. (1960). *Cancer Res.* **20,** 351.

Fishman, M. (1961). *J. Exp. Med.* **114,** 837.

Freeman, C. B., Harris, R., Geary, C. G., Leyland, M. J., MacIver, J. E. and Delamore, I. W. (1973). *Brit. med. J.* **4,** 571.

Freund, J. (1956). *Adv. Tuberc. Res.* **7,** 130.

Freundlich, E. and Suprun, H. (1969). *Israel J. Med. Sci.* **5,** 108.

Ghose, T. and Nigam, S. P. (1972a). *Cancer* **29,** 1398.

Ghose, T., Norvell, S. T., Guclu, A., Cameron, D., Bodurtha, A. and MacDonald, A. S. (1972b). *Brit. med. J.* **3,** 495.

Goldenberg, E. J. and Brandes, L. J. (1972). *Clin. Res.* **20,** 947.

Golub, S. H., Svedmyr, E. A. J., Hewetson, J. F., Klein, G. and Singh, S. (1972). *Int. J. Cancer* **10,** 157.

Golub, S. H., Roth, J. A., Forsythe, A. and Morton, D. L. (1976). *Bibl. Haemat.* **43,** 270.

Gormsen, H. (1955). *Acta. Path. Microbiol. Scand.* **Suppl. 111,** 117.

Graber, H. and Takacs, L. and Vedrody, K. (1976). *Lancet* **2,** 1248.

Graham, J. B. and Graham, R. M. (1959). *Surg. Gynec. Obstet.* **109,** 131.

Grant, R. M., Mackie, R. M., Cochran, A. J., Murray, E. L., Hoyle, D. E. and Ross, C. E. (1974). *Lancet* **2,** 1096.

Gutterman, J. U., Mavligit, G., McBride, C., Frei, E. III and Hersh, E. M. (1973). *Cancer* **32,** 321.

Gutterman, J. U., McBride, C., Freireich, E. J., Mavligit, G., Frei, E. III and Hersh, E. M. (1973). *Lancet* **1,** 1208.

Gutterman, J. U., Mavligit, G., McBride, C., Frei, E. III and Hersh, E. M. (1974). *In* "Immunological Aspects of Neoplasia". Year Book Medical Publishers, Chicago.

Gutterman, J. U., Rodriguez, V., Mavligit, G., Burgess, M. A., Gehan, E., Hersh, E. M., McCredie, K. B., Reed, R., Smith, T., Bodey, G. P. and Freireich, E. J. (1974). *Lancet* **2,** 1405.

Halle-Pannenko, O., Bourut, C. and Kamel, M. (1976). *Cancer Immunol. Immunother.* **1,** 17.

Halpern, B., Biozzi, G., Stiffel, C. and Mouton, D. (1966). *Nature* **212,** 853.

Halpern, B. (1975). "Corynebacterium parvum." Plenum Press, London.

Hardy, D. A., Ling, N. R. and Walling, J. (1970). *Nature* **227,** 723.

Harris, J. E. and Sinkovics, J. G. (1970). "Immunology of Malignant Disease." Mosby, St. Louis.

Hersh, E. M., Gutterman, J. U. and Mavligit, G. M. (1974). *Cancer Treatment Reviews* **1,** 65.

Hibbs, J. B. Jr., Lambert, L. H. and Remington, J. S. (1972). *Nature (New Biol.)* **235,** 48.

Hirshaut, Y., Pinsky, C., Marquardt, H., Oettgen, H. F. (1977). *Proc. Amer. Ass. Cancer Res.* **14**, 109.

Hiu, I. J. (1972). *Nature (New Biol.)* **238**, 241.

Hollinshead, A. C. and Stewart, T. H. M. (1977). *In* "Proceedings of the Third International Symposium on Cancer Detection and Prevention".

Holmes, E. C. and Golub, S. H. (1976). *J. Thorac. Cardiovasc. Surg.* **71**, 161.

Hopper, D. G., Pimm, M. V. and Baldwin, R. W. (1975). *Brit. J. Cancer* **32**, 345.

Horn, L. and Horn, H. L. (1971). *Lancet* **2**, 466.

Hunt, J. S., Silverstein, M. J., Sparks, F. C., Haskell, C. M., Pilch, Y. H. and Morton, D. L. (1973). *Lancet* **2**, 820.

Ikonopisov, R. L. (1970). *Brit. Med. J.* **2**, 752.

Ikonopisov, R. L. (1972). *Tumori* **58**, 121.

Israel, L. and Halpern, B. (1972). *Nouv. Presse. Med.* **1**, 1.

Israel, L. (1975). *In* "Corynebacterium parvum" (Halpern, B., Ed.) 389. Plenum Press, London.

Jacobsen, C. (1934). *Arch. f. Derm. u. Syph.* **169**, 562.

Johnson, R. K., Houchens, D. P., Gaston, M. R. and Goldin, A. (1975). *Cancer Chemother. Rep.* **59(4)**, 697.

Jurczyk-Procyk, S., Martin, M., Dubouch, P., Gheroghiu, M., Economides, F., Khalil, A. and Rappaport, H. (1976). *Cancer Immunol. Immunother.* (In Press.)

Klein, G., Sjögren, H. O., Klein, E. and Hellström, K. E. (1966). *Cancer Res.* **20**, 1561.

Klein, E. (1969). *Cancer Res.* **29**, 2351.

Lamensans, A., Stiffel, C., Mollier, F., Laurent, M., Mouton, D. and Biozzi, G. (1968). *Rev. Franc. Etud. Clin. Biol.* **13**, 773.

Lawrence, H. S. (1955). *J. Clin. Invest.* **34**, 219.

Lawrence, H. S. (1969). *Adv. Immunol.,* **11**, 195.

Levin, A. S., Spitler, L. E., Stites, D. P. and Fudenberg, H. H. (1970). *Proc. nat. Acad. Sci.* **67**, 821.

Levin, A. S., Byers, V. S., Fudenberg, H. H., Wybran, J., Hackett, A. J. and Johnston, J. O. (1975). *J. Clin. Invest.* **55**, 487.

Lewis, P. A. and Loomis, D. (1924). *J. exp. Med.* **40**, 503.

Lewisohn, R., Leuchtenberger, C., Leuchtenberger, R., Laszlo, D. and Block, K. (1941). *Cancer Res.* **1**, 799.

Littman, B. H., Meltzer, M. S., Cleveland, R. P., Zbar, B. and Rapp, H. (1973). *J. nat. Cancer Inst.* **51**, 1627.

Mackaness, G. B., Lagrange, P. H. and Ishibushi, T. (1974). *J. exp. Med.* **139**, 1540.

Mackie, R. M., Jackson, A. M., Ogg, L. J. and Cochran, A. J. *Pigment Cell* **4**, In Press.

Maeda, H. (1973). "Immunopotentiation." Ciba Symposium, London.

Maisin, J., Pourbaix, V. and Caeymeax, D. (1938). *C. rend. Soc. Biol.* **127**, 1477.

Malek-Mansour, S., Castermans-Elias, S. and Lapiere, C. M. (1973). *Dermatol. (Basel)* **146**, 156.

Mannick, J. A. and Egdahl, R. H. (1964). *J. Clin. Invest.* **43**, 2166.

Mantovani. A. and Spreafico, F. (1975). *Europ. J. Cancer* **11**, 537.

Marsh, B., Flynn, L. and Enneking, W. (1972). *J. Bone and Joint Surg.* **54A**, 1367.

Martin, D. S., Hayworth, P., Fugmann, R. A., English, R. and McNeil, H. W. (1964). *Cancer Res.* **24**, 652.

Mathé, G., Loc, T. B. and Bernard, J. (1958). *C. rend. Acad. Sci. Paris* **246**, 1626.

Mathé, G., Amiel, J. L., Schwarzenberg, L., Schneider, M., Cattan, A., Schlumberger, J. R., Hayat, M. and deVassal, F. (1963). *Rev. Franc. d'Etudes clin. et biol.* **13,** 454.

Mathé, G., Schwarzenberg, L., Amiel, J. L., Cattan, A. and Schlumberger, J. R. (1967). *Cancer Res.* **27,** 2542.

Mathé, G., Amiel, J. L., Schwarzenberg, L., Schneider, M., Cattan, A., Schlumberger, J. R., Hayat, M. and deVassal, F. (1969). *Lancet* **1,** 697.

Mathé, G. (1972). *Ann. Inst. Pasteur Paris,* **122,** 855.

Mathé, G. (1975). *Nouv. Presse Med.* **4,** 1333.

Mathé, G. (1976). *Cancer Immunol. Immunother.* **1,** 3.

Matsaniotis, N. (1967). *Acta Paediatr. Scand. (Suppl.)* **172,** 146.

Medical Research Council Leukaemia Committee (1971). *Brit. med. J.* **4,** 189.

Medical Research Council (1972). *Bull. W.H.O.* **46,** 371.

Mellman, W. J. and Wetton, R. (1963). *J. Lab. clin. Invest.* **61,** 453.

Milton, G. W. and Lan Brown, M. M. (1966). *Aust. N.Z. J. Surg.* **35,** 286.

Morton, D. L., Eilber, F. R., Malmgren, R. A. and Wood, W. C. (1970). *Surgery* **68,** 158.

Morton, D. L., Eilber, F. R., Holmes, E. C., Hunt, J. S., Ketcham, A. S., Silverstein, M. J. and Sparks, F. C. (1974). *Ann. Surg.* **180,** 635.

Morton, D. L., Eilber, F. R., Holmes, E. C., Sparks, F. C. and Ramming, K. P. (1976). *Cancer Immunol. Immunother.* **1,** 93.

McCarthy, W. H., Cotton, G., Carlon, A., Milton, G. W. and Kossard, S. (1973). *Cancer* **32,** 97.

McGrath, I. T. (1975). *Int. J. Cancer* **13,** 839.

McIlmurray, M. B., Embleton, M. J., Reeves, W. G., Langman, M. J. S. and Deane, M. (1977). *Brit. med. J.* **1,** 540.

McKhann, C. F., Hendrickson, C. G., Spitler, L. E., Gunnarsson, A., Banerjee, D. and Nelson, W. R. (1975). *Cancer* **35,** 514.

McKneally, M. F., Mavor, C. and Kausel, H. W. (1976). *Lancet* **1,** 377.

Nadler, S. H. and Moore, G. E. (1965). *Surg. Forum* **16,** 229.

Nagy, I., Jeno, A. and Koszuro, M. (1971). *Arch. Ital. Patolg. Clin. Tumor* **14,** 29.

Nathanson, L., Hall, T. C. and Farber, S. (1967). *Cancer* **20,** 650.

Nathanson, L. (1972). *Cancer Chemoth. Rep.* **56,** 659.

Nauts, H. C., Swift, W. E. and Coley, B. L. (1946). *Cancer Res.* **6,** 205.

Nauts, H. C., Fowler, G. A. and Bogatko, F. H. (1953). *Acta. med. Scnad.* **145,** (Suppl.) 276.

Ngu, V. A. (1967). *Brit. med. J.* **1,** 345.

Old, L. J., Clark, D. A. and Benacerraf, B. (1959). *Nature* **184,** 291.

Old, L. J., Benacerraf, B., Clarke, D. A., Carswell, E. A. and Stockert, E. (1961). *Cancer Res.* **21,** 1281.

Oon, C. J., Butterworth, C., Elliott, P., Hobbs, J. R., McLeod, B., Rosengurk, N. and Westbury, G. (1975). *Behring Inst. Mitt.* **56,** 223.

Order, S. E., Kirkman, R. and Knapp, R. (1974). *Cancer* **34,** 175.

Pilch, Y. H., Fritze, D. and Kern, D. H. (1975). *Behring Inst. Mitt.* **56,** 184.

Pines, A. (1976). *Lancet* **1,** 380.

Pinsky, C., Hirshaut, Y. and Oettgen, H. (1972). *Proc. Amer. Assoc. Cancer Res.* **13,** 21.

Pressman, D. and Korngold, L. (1953). *Cancer* **6,** 619.

Pressman, D., Yagi, Y. and Hiramoto, R. A. (1958). *Arch. Allerg. Appl. Immunol.* **12,** 125.

Ramming, K. P. and Pilch, Y. H. (1970). *Science* **168**, 492.
Rapapport, F. T. and Lawrence, H. S. (1975). *In* "Cancer and Transplantation" (Murphy, G. P., Ed.). Grune and Stratton, New York.
Reed, R. C., Gutterman, J. U., Mavligit, G. M., Burgess, A. A. and Hersh, E. M. (1975). *In* "Corynebacterium parvum" (Halpern, B., Ed.) 349. Plenum Press, London.
Ribi, E., Anacker, R. L. and Barclay, W. R. (1971). *Infect. Dis.* **123**, 528.
Ribi, E., Larson, C. and Wicht, W. (1966). *J. Bact.* **91**, 975.
Rojas, A. F., Mickiewicz, E., Peierstein, J. N., Glait, H. and Olivari, A. J. (1976). *Lancet* **1**, 211.
Rosenthal, S. R., Crispen, R. G., Thorne, M. G. *et al.* (1972). *J. Amer. med. Ass.* **222**, 1543.
Rosenthal, M., Trabert, U. and Muller, W. (1976). *Lancet* **1**, 369.
Ruuskanen, O., Remes, M., Makela, A. L., Isomaki, H. and Toivanen, A. (1976). *Lancet* **2**, 958.
Sabbadini, E. and Sehon, A. H. (1967). *Internat. Arch. Allerg. Appl. Immunol.* **32**, 55.
Sadowski, J. M. and Rapp, F. (1975). *Proc. Soc. exp. Biol. Med.* **149**, 219.
Salaman, M. H. (1969). *Antibiotica et Chemotherapia* **15**, 393.
Scanlon, E. F., Hawkins, R. A., Fox, W. W. and Smith, W. S. (1965). *Cancer* **18**, 782.
Sensenig, D. M., Rossi, N. P. and Ehrenhaft, J. L. (1963). *Surg. Gynec. Obstet.* **116**, 229.
Serrou, B., Dubois, J. B., Meiss, L. and Romieu, C. (1975). *Panminerva Med.* **17**, 182.
Serrou, B., Michel, H., Dubois, J. R. and Serre, A. (1975). *Biomed.* **23**, 236.
Shibata, H. R., Jerry, L. M., Lewis, M. G., Mansell, P. W., Capek, A. and Marquis, A. (1975). *In* "Proceedings of International Conference on immunotherapy of cancer". New York Academy of Science.
Simmons, R. L. and Rios, A. (1971). *Science* **174**, 591.
Smith, S. E. and Scott, J. (1972). *Brit. J. Cancer* **26**, 361.
Sokal, J. E., Aungst, C. W. and Grace, J. T. Jr. (1973). *N.Y.J. Med.* **73**, 1180.
Southam, C. M. (1961). *Cancer Res.* **21**, 302.
Southam, C. M., Marcove, R. C., Levin, A. G., Buchsbaum, H. J. and Mike, V. (1973). "Seventh National Cancer Conference." 91. Lippincott, Philadelphia.
Sparks, F. C., Silverstein, M. J., Hunt, J. S., Haskell, C. M., Pilch, Y. H. and Morton, D. L. (1973). *New Engl. J. Med.* **18**, 827.
Starr, S. and Berkovitch, S. (1964). *New Engl. J. Med.* **270**, 386.
Stern, K. (1971). *Israel J. med. Sci.* **7**, 42.
Stewart, T. H. M. and Tolnai, G. (1969). *Cancer* **24**, 201.
Stjernswärd, J. and Levin, A. (1971). *Cancer* **28**, 628.
Sumner, W. C. and Foraker, K. G. (1960). *Cancer* **13**, 79.
Symes, M. O., Riddell, A. G., Immelmann, E. J. and Terblanche, J. (1968). *Lancet* **1**, 1054.
Symes, M. O., Riddell, A. G., Feneley, R. C. and Tribe, C. R. (1973a). *Birt. J. Cancer* **28**, (Suppl. 1), 276.
Symes, M. O. and Riddell, A. G. (1973b). *Brit. J. Surg.* **60**, 176.
Symoens, J. (1976). "Levamisole Technical Review." Janssen Pharmaceuticals, Beerse, Belgium.
Takakura, K. (1975). Proceedings 34th Meeting Japanese Cancer Association.
Takita, H. (1970). *J. Thorac. Cardiovasc. Surg.* **59**, 642.
Teimourian, B. and McCune, W. S. (1963). *Amer. Surg.* **29**, 515.

Terry, W. (1978) Immunotherapy of Cancer: Present status of trials in man. Raven Press, New York.
Tripodi, D., Parks, L. C. and Brugmans, J. (1973). *New Engl. J. Med.* **289**, 354.
Vanholder, R. and Van Hove, W. (1977). *Lancet* **1**, 100.
Veltman, L. L., Kern, D. H. and Pilch, Y. H. (1974). *Cell. Immunol.* **13**, 367.
Vogler, W. R. and Chan, Y.-K. (1974). *Lancet* **2**, 128.
vonPirquet, C. (1908). *Deutsche Med. Woch.* **34**, 1297.
Ward, H. W. C. (1976). *Lancet* **1**, 594.
Warner, J. (1966). *Brit. J. Dermatol.* **78**, 549.
Watanabe, T., Tanka, K. and Hagiwara, Y. (1969). *Acta. Path. Jap.* **19**, 395.
Watkins, E., Ogata, Y., Anderson, L. L., Watkins, E. III and Waters, M. F. (1971). *Nature (New Biol.)* **231**, 85.
Watkins, S. M. (1971). *Brit. med. J.* **1**, 492.
Wedderburn, N. (1970). *Lancet* **2**, 1114.
Weiss, D. W. (1972). *Nat. Cancer Inst. Monogr.* **35**, 157.
Williams, I. A. (1976). *Lancet* **1**, 1080.
Willoughby, H., Latour, J. P. A., Tabah, E. J. and Shibata, H. R. (1970). *Amer. J. Obstet. Gynec.* **108**, 889.
Witebsky, E., Rose, N. R. and Shulman, S. (1956). *Cancer Res.* **16**, 831.
Woodruff, M. F. A. and Nolan, B. (1963). *Lancet* **2**, 426.
Woodruff, M. F. A. and Boak, J. L. (1966). *Brit. J. Cancer* **20**, 343.
Woodruff, M. F. A. and Dunbar, N. (1973). "Immunopotentiation." 287. Elsevier-Excerpta Medica, North Holland, Amsterdam.
Woodruff, M. F. A., Clunie, G. J. A., McBride, W. H., McCormack, R. J. M., Walbaum, P. R. and James, K. (1975). *In* "Corynebacterium parvum" (Halpern, B., Ed.) 383. Plenum Press, London.
Yonemoto, R. H. and Terasaki, P. (1972). *Cancer* **30**, 1438.
Zbar, B. and Rapp, H. J. (1974). *Cancer* **34**, 1532.
Zbar, B., Ribi, E., Meyer, T., Azuma, I. and Rapp, H. J. (1974). *J. nat. Cancer Inst.* **52**, 1571.
Zbar, B., Smith, H., Bast, R. and Rapp, J. (1975). *Behring Inst. Mitt.* **56**, 35.

Index